Stop Diabetes Now

AVERY

a member of

Penguin Group (USA) Inc.

New York

Stop Diabetes Now

 A Groundbreaking Program for Controlling Your Disease and Staying Healthy

WILLIAM T. CEFALU, M.D.

A Lynn Sonberg Book

Catherine M. Champagne, Ph.D., R.D.
Nutrition and Exercise Editor

Published by the Penguin Group
Penguin Group (USA) Inc., 375 Hudson Street, New York, New York 10014, USA • Penguin Group (Canada),
90 Eglinton Avenue East, Suite 700, Toronto, Ontario M4P 2Y3, Canada (a division of Pearson Canada Inc.) •
Penguin Books Ltd, 80 Strand, London WC2R 0RL, England • Penguin Ireland, 25 St Stephen's Green,
Dublin 2, Ireland (a division of Penguin Books Ltd) • Penguin Group (Australia), 250 Camberwell Road,
Camberwell, Victoria 3124, Australia (a division of Pearson Australia Group Pty Ltd) • Penguin Books India Pvt Ltd,
11 Community Centre, Panchsheel Park, New Delhi–110 017, India • Penguin Group (NZ), 67 Apollo Drive,
Rosedale, North Shore 0632, New Zealand (a division of Pearson New Zealand Ltd) • Penguin
Books (South Africa) (Pty) Ltd, 24 Sturdee Avenue, Rosebank, Johannesburg 2196, South Africa

Penguin Books Ltd, Registered Offices: 80 Strand, London WC2R 0RL, England

Most Avery books are available at special quantity discounts for bulk purchase for sales promotions,
premiums, fund-raising, and educational needs. Special books or book excerpts also can be created to fit specific
needs. For details, write Penguin Group (USA) Inc. Special Markets, 375 Hudson Street, New York, NY 10014.

Library of Congress Cataloging-in-Publication Data
Cefalu, William T.
Stop diabetes now: a groundbreaking program for controlling
your disease and staying healthy/William T. Cefalu.
p.   cm.
ISBN 978-1-58333-308-2
1. Diabetes—Popular works.   I. Title.
RC660.4.C438   2008   2008006373
616.4'62—dc22

Printed in the United States of America
1   3   5   7   9   10   8   6   4   2

Neither the publisher nor the author is engaged in rendering professional advice or services to the individual reader. The ideas, procedures, and suggestions contained in this book are not intended as a substitute for consulting with your physician. All matters regarding your health require medical supervision. Neither the author nor the publisher shall be liable or responsible for any loss or damage allegedly arising from any information or suggestion in this book.

All efforts have been made to ensure the accuracy of the information contained in this book as of the date published. The author and publisher expressly disclaim responsibility for any adverse effects arising from the use or application of the information contained herein.

The recipes contained in this book are to be followed exactly as written. The publisher is not responsible for your specific health or allergy needs that may require medical supervision. The publisher is not responsible for any adverse reactions to the recipes contained in this book.

While the author has made every effort to provide accurate telephone numbers and Internet addresses at the time of publication, neither the publisher nor the author assumes any responsibility for errors, or for changes that occur after publication. Further, the publisher does not have any control over and does not assume any responsibility for author or third-party websites or their content.

Acknowledgments

WHERE DOES ONE BEGIN to thank all the individuals responsible for helping directly or indirectly with the creation of this book? I have to look no further than my wife, Liz, and two wonderful sons, Christopher and Jonathan, for the roles they have played. Clearly, to have the time and drive to write such a book simply means I have been provided a wonderful family structure that has allowed for personal and professional growth. My work is incredibly important to me, yet I can't imagine anyone being able to concentrate on work if his home situation is not stable or satisfying. I have my wife to thank for that, since she has been the most important part of my life and has created a family situation for which I consider myself the luckiest guy in the world! More important, my wife deserves a tremendous amount of credit for "walking the walk"—that is, adhering to the lifestyle and nutritional advice in this book. For our family, it is a major objective and a way of life!

Like many other families, ours has social activities centered around food and drink, which are of course an important part of entertaining and family life. Years ago, my wife and I were on the same "treadmill" many families were on, trying to provide activities for our young children that sitting down and enjoying meals together was sacrificed for a "quick bite" here or a "drive through" there. But happily, both of us recognized long ago the value of a healthy lifestyle, including adequate nutrition and plenty of exercise, not only for our individual health, but for the health of the family unit. To this end my wife has strived for years now to cook just about every night with significant planning and preparation, experimenting with different cooking styles and flavors. Her meals are living proof that one can eat foods that are both delicious and nutritionally balanced. These family meals are sacred and we allow no interference from phone calls or TV. Best of all, over time these principles have been instilled in my two sons who, as young adults, now have nutritional habits and exercise routines that I am proud of! The fact that we emphasized a healthful lifestyle seems to be paying dividends. So, I owe a tremendous amount of credit to my wife who made this happen.

I would also like to give credit to an individual who I have grown to respect not only as a colleague, but as a friend. Dr. Catherine Champagne played an important role in guiding the information in the nutritional chapters. Dr. Champagne's research areas currently concentrate on studies that include dietary counseling and/or dietary intake assessment of subjects. She supervises a team of dietitians, programmers, and other support personnel and her areas of expertise include food composition, menu design for specialized nutrient targets, dietary assessment, counseling strategies for chronic disease conditions, obesity, and cardiovascular disease. Her interests are women and children's health, diet for weight loss and chronic disease, Mediterranean diet approaches for reduction of cardiovascular disease risk, physical activity, and nutritional assessment of diverse populations. Dr. Champagne was involved in the initial conceptualization of the Diabetes Prevention Project and Look AHEAD Trial. Additionally, she was instrumental in the development of the menus used in the DASH and DASH-Sodium trials. The Pennington Biomedical Research Center's nutrient database was the database of choice in the DASH trials, and Dr. Champagne manages those activities at the center. So, as you read the nutritional chapters and chapters for recipes, take great comfort that the information there has been reviewed and provided by another person who "walks the walk."

Thank you also to Maggie Greenwood-Robinson for pulling together research studies, organizing the contents, and helping me put into words the scientific information that can help so many people stop the progression of their diabetes.

To Lynn Sonberg I give credit and thanks for making this book a reality. She guided the process superbly, offered wise counsel, and kept me focused throughout the writing.

Realize that in writing this book, I am simply breaking down the science from researchers who, over the years, have made incredible advances in understanding the causes of diabetes and in helping individuals live better lives if they have diabetes. Research is not an easy job. Obtaining money for research is not getting any easier. The research cited in this book is the summary of years of dedicated efforts for diabetes researchers around the world, and they should be given the credit for the messages in this book.

Finally, I have to give credit to major governing agencies whose main mission is to stem this epidemic. These include agencies like the National Institutes of Health, which funded through tax dollars the landmark trials mentioned in this book. I also have to acknowledge the American Diabetes Association and Juvenile Diabetes Foundation for funding research efforts. In addition, the American Diabetes Association has provided guidelines and standards of care to which physicians and patients should strive to adhere. These guidelines are based on evidence-based research and are emphasized over and over again in this book.

So, in closing, you can see that this book is a group effort and I am privileged to be considered the "messenger."

Contents

Introduction: The Solution You Need Now   1

Part 1: Diabetes Today: Overview of an Epidemic

1 Understanding Diabetes and How We Can Stop It   9

2 Beware of Metabolic Syndrome and Prediabetes   21

3 The Good and Bad News about Complications   34

Part 2: A Lifestyle Prescription for Preventing and Managing Diabetes

4 Making the Most of Your Food   61

5 Meal Plans and Recipes to Prevent or Manage Diabetes   92

6   The Promise of Complementary Therapy   131

7   Exercising Your Options   156

8   Glucose Testing Made Pain-Free and Easy   175

9   Keeping the Momentum: Reap the Benefits of Outside Support   187

Part 3: Medical Management

10   Optimizing Your Antidiabetes Medications   203

11   Using Insulin: Not the Pain It Used to Be   217

Appendices

Appendix A: Glossary   227

Appendix B: Stretching Exercises and Guidelines   241

Appendix C: Resources   245

Appendix D: References   251

Index   256

Introduction
The Solution You Need Now

HOW WOULD YOU LIKE TO STOP THE PROGRESSION OF YOUR DIABETES?

If you are among the more than twenty-one million people in this country who have diabetes, I am giving you the hopeful message that you can stop this disease from overtaking your health and your life.

Yes, diabetes is an epidemic. If ignored, it can devastate lives and families. Now more than ever, there is much you can do to prevent it, or halt its progress. Through scientific research, we now have information on diet, exercise, glucose control, and medication that you can use on a day-to-day basis to manage your diabetes and its risk factors most effectively.

For example, we now have landmark research that defines the lifestyle changes, such as diet and exercise, required to effectively stop diabetes, and even to prevent it. In this book, I will outline for you the very same diet used in this research that helped people lose approximately 5 percent of their body weight, plus drop their risk of developing diabetes by approximately 58 percent.

I will also present the latest facts about nutritional supplements that claim to treat diabetes. It is important to know what works and what does not work. At this time, the findings regarding most over-the-counter supplements are more promising than proven. I will tell you what we do know, what we don't know, and what still needs to be learned in this area.

Exercise is also a vital part of the prescription for stopping diabetes. But you would be surprised at the amount of exercise you actually need to benefit your diabetes. We know unequivocally from major research studies that just a very moderate amount of exercise—about twenty minutes a day—is instrumental in changing the course of this disease.

If you are like many diabetics, you may resist or delay blood sugar monitoring because it has traditionally involved the painful process of pricking your finger to draw blood. Yet not monitoring your blood sugar and not knowing your levels can be extremely detrimental to your health. Fortunately, there are promising devices on the market that minimize pain and discomfort, including implantable glucose monitors, and you will learn about them here.

We also know that certain prescription medications show great promise in the prevention of diabetes, thanks to landmark research in this area. Along those lines, there are also several classes of new drugs available, and now we have newer agents that work very differently from any drug available in the past. One class of agents is called "incretins," and they not only control blood glucose, but may also help you control your weight. The good news, too, is that they work well with other drugs you may take.

Why This Book Is Different

Go into any bookstore and you'll find no end of titles on diabetes. What I'm offering is the very latest in diabetes research and how to apply it to your day-to-day life. It is a truly integrative approach to controlling diabetes. What that means is a program that intentionally uses conventional medical treatments alongside other scientifically proven practices involving diet, supplements, and exercise to better your condition—plus one that emphasizes the very crux of diabetes management, "metabolic" control. I define "metabolic control" as one that includes gaining tighter control of your blood sugar, as well as improving your blood pressure and your cholesterol levels.

Tighter blood sugar control, in particular, is vitally important. Based on the progression of diabetes and the fact that the oral medications may not control diabetes for many people, I feel that more people with type 2 diabetes should use insulin earlier in addition to managing their diets more carefully and making lifestyle changes, since the very latest research bears this out. Don't let that scare you—let it encourage you, since insulin is a known, powerful medicine that essentially is replacing what the body is lacking. When you begin to keep your blood sugar within a certain range and closer to that seen for an individual without diabetes, you can stop diabetes in its tracks.

By "range," I mean to keep your average glucose in line with the current recommended guidelines, as measured by A1c, an important test that measures your average blood glucose level, as currently suggested by the American Diabetes Association. Current recommendations are to keep this value below 7 percent. However, you may have heard that this value was questioned by a recent study. Specifically, over the recent past, a federally funded trial called the Action to Control Cardiovascular Risk in Diabetes (ACCORD) study found that intensively reducing blood sugar below those guidelines caused harm in high-risk patients with type 2 diabetes. In this study, patients were considered "high risk" if they had vascular disease or at least two of the following cardiovascular risk factors for vascular disease, including high blood pressure, high cholesterol, obesity, and smoking. It should be noted that the patient population studied and the means for achieving the tight glycemic control are not commonly encountered in the majority of primary care practices. Thus, the findings may not change the practice of the vast majority of diabetes cases. As such, important and additional new information was also supplied by investigators of another large-scale, randomized clinical trial addressing a similar question of whether more intensive glucose control would improve clinical outcomes in patients with diabetes. This data comes from the ADVANCE trial and the results provide no confirmation of the concern reported from the ACCORD study regarding intensive glycemic control and heart disease. As stated, doctors and patients should feel reassured that this concern has not been found in the interim results from ADVANCE. Clearly, we need to await more definitive analyses and reports from both studies before drawing final conclusions, but until then, we should adhere to the currently recommended guidelines for glycemic control.

As for medical therapy, I firmly believe that insulin and other medicines absolutely do work hand in hand with nutrition, exercise, and other lifestyle changes. In the approach to stopping diabetes outlined in this book, the whole is definitely greater than the sum of its parts, as the familiar adage goes. There is no one single solution to blood sugar control; it takes an intensive combination of research-backed approaches—and that is the difference I bring you in this book.

A Plan That Breaks the Science into Easy, Manageable Steps

As a physician, I chose to specialize in diabetes because it is a condition that affects all organ systems, and thus gave me an opportunity to do research in any area of the body I wanted. For nearly two decades, I have been an investigator involved in evaluating novel therapies for individuals with diabetes and studies of the risk factors for diabetes, including obesity, high cholesterol, and high blood pressure, and have worked on ways to reduce their impact. These studies have been supported by the National Institutes of Health (NIH), American Diabetes Association, and major pharmaceutical companies. In addition, I have been a clinician actively involved in patient care. As a result, I have a scientifically based understanding of the most current information about how lifestyle affects the development of diabetes, and how you can prevent or manage it most effectively. I have hands-on experience in day-to-day diabetes and obesity management and will share proven strategies to help you succeed in making the difficult lifestyle changes necessary to achieve weight loss and/or weight maintenance, normal cholesterol levels, and healthy blood pressure.

I draw on my background to provide you with the very latest treatments and approaches that will make a dramatic difference in your life if you have diabetes, or if you are at risk for it. In fact, I take a "translational" approach to educating you about diabetes. Simply put, I will decipher the science for you and put it into practical terms you can use right away. Normally, it may take many years before research findings published in medical journals become common practice by providers. I'm going to speed up that process for you and give you information you and your doctor can use today. I will discuss the suggested standards of care for diabetes management. For example, major organizations such as the American Diabetes Association have provided specific recommendations to follow if you have diabetes so as to prevent and delay the complications of diabetes, but many individuals with diabetes are not aware of these guidelines. This book contains the very latest scientifically proven recommendations, organized into a doable plan, for controlling diabetes and halting its complications.

Live Better

I wrote this book for people who are at risk for developing diabetes and want to avoid it; for people who are struggling with the disease and want to feel better; and for the families who love them. Some of you are experiencing complications from diabetes that have reached a critical level. Now the disease is seriously affecting the quality of your life. But do not despair. In the twenty-plus years I have been researching diabetes and treating patients, I have seen the results of alterations in diet, lifestyle, and medication—powerful therapy that can help prevent further decline and bring you undeniable improvements in your health.

Diabetes can not only be prevented; with proper diet, lifestyle, and sometimes the right medication, the progression of diabetes to the devastating complications may be stopped, and I will say that over and over again. This was only a dream years ago, but now it is reality. New research, new drugs, new forms of insulin, and less painful ways to give insulin have yielded treatments that can begin this process for most patients.

By using the plan outlined in this book, you have the potential to stop your own diabetes and the march of its potentially deadly complications. Most patients, particularly those with type 2 diabetes, begin to live fuller, healthier lives when they follow this plan. Some benefit dramatically from simple dietary changes. Others learn how to integrate lifestyle with medications, and enjoy a long life free of the complications of diabetes or better manage the complications if they exist already.

I want to say at the start that if you have diabetes, nothing in this book will make it go away and reverse your condition. The fact is that physiologically, once you have diabetes, you have it for life. This does not mean you can't control it, lower your blood sugar, or live a full, healthy life. In fact, quite the opposite is true! There is no question that diabetes *is* a progressive disease—but not if you take aggressive charge of it. Again, I need to emphasize that, based on what we know about the natural history of type 2 diabetes, over time, unless you and your doctor take matters into your own hands, accessing the latest nutritional knowledge, exercise recommendations, and medical treatments, blood sugars most likely will get worse. Treatments must keep pace with the disease progression. In other words, this book is providing for you the practical advice that you need to bypass the chain of diabetic consequences.

Whenever this route of positive action is taken, I see more and more patients who look, act, and live as if they did not have the disease. The plan outlined in this book provides *you* with the day-to-day information you need to halt the progressive nature of the disease. You do not have to experience physical decline and loss of health. The plan described in this book is one you can live with, so that you can enjoy a long life free of the complications of diabetes. For many of you, it will mean an improved level of health that maybe you didn't think was realistically attainable.

This is an exciting time of hope and promise if you have diabetes, or are at risk for it. By applying the science in this book, and taking advantage of the latest developments in diabetes medicine, you can feel better, live better, and enjoy quality of life every day.

Don't you think you should begin right now?

Part 1

Diabetes Today: Overview of an Epidemic

Understanding Diabetes and How We Can Stop It

IF YOUR DOCTOR HAS JUST TOLD YOU that you have diabetes, you're probably reeling with shock and filled with questions. What does this mean? How will this change my life? How will this affect my longevity?

Take a deep breath and relax. I have some encouraging words for you: it is within your control to recapture your health, or better yet, improve it. This is a disease that, to a startling degree, is treatable and manageable. What it takes is a comprehensive, multipronged approach, using the most up-to-date nutritional know-how, the latest medicines, the most current glucose-monitoring methods, and the best advice on exercise and other lifestyle changes. None of these works without the other—remember that treatment must be intensive and integrative—and all of these approaches go hand in hand if you want to successfully stop diabetes and its complications, including serious damage to the eyes, nerves, heart, kidneys, and blood vessels.

You can change your life and prevent and better manage diabetes. Further, you can significantly delay complications if you already have diabetes. No one is a victim here.

A good example of this positive way of looking at diabetes is Terry, who had come to our clinic for treatment. You would never know she had diabetes. Terry was diagnosed with type 1 diabetes twenty-one years earlier, while she was in high school. When her doctor told her she had the disease, she felt as though her world was "crashing in" around her.

"I didn't think I could do the things my friends were doing or enjoy things in life like pizza and snacks at parties," she told me. "My friends even seemed to treat me differently, as they didn't understand."

Wisely, her doctor recommend that she attend diabetic camps during the summer, where she lived day to day with other people her age, also with diabetes.

"The camps were great and showed to me that I am no different from anyone else. I just have diabetes and learned that if I controlled it, I could live a normal healthy life."

Terry has managed her diabetes throughout the years with frequent blood sugar checks and multiple injections of insulin. Not long ago, she gave birth to her first son after carefully managing her diabetes through pregnancy. With regard to her child, she states, "I now have another reason to take care of myself."

Proof That You Can Stop Diabetes

Throughout this book, you will learn what Terry already knows: how to prevent and manage your diabetes through adequate control of your blood sugar. This has been shown to significantly reduce the progression to complications such as eye disease, kidney disease, and nerve disease, in both type 1 and type 2 diabetes. Specifically, evidence for the importance of blood sugar control comes from the Diabetes Control and Complications Trial (DCCT), the largest, most comprehensive type 1 diabetes trial ever conducted, with results reported in 1993 and followed up in 2005.

For example, according to a key finding of the DCCT study, if you maintain blood glucose levels as close to normal as possible, there are startling benefits, even if you have a history of poor blood sugar control. Because the study evaluated individuals with type 1 diabetes, the change in therapy had to do with an "intensive" insulin regimen (multiple injections daily) as opposed to "conventional" (two injections). The initial findings in this study demonstrated that the risk of diabetic nerve damage (neuropathy), diabetic kidney disease, and diabetic eye disease were remarkably reduced with improvement in blood glucose. After this study followed the patients for many years, the researchers observed that this brand of "intensive therapy" reduced the risk of having heart or blood vessel problems by 42 percent. It reduced the chance of having a heart attack, stroke, or dying from cardiovascular disease by 57 percent. These findings are truly remarkable.

Similar findings were seen for people with type 2 diabetes in the United Kingdom Prospective Diabetes Study (UKPDS), the largest clinical study of type 2 diabetes ever attempted. It showed that the life-threatening complications of type 2 diabetes, including heart disease, stroke, and early kidney damage, as well as diabetic eye disease, can be significantly reduced by tighter blood glucose control and better blood pressure control (in diabetic patients with hypertension).

To achieve adequate glucose control, according to the lessons learned from these landmark studies, you should do the following:

- Establish a support system with a health-care team, make routine visits to your team, and know your numbers for the suggested level of blood glucose, blood pressure, and cholesterol.
- Implement an appropriate nutritional plan and physical activity into your treatment program. These are "cornerstones" of therapy and should be designed so that they can easily fit into your daily life.
- Work with your physician to design a schedule of blood glucose testing that is appropriate for your condition and allows you to either adjust your insulin or oral medication.
- If you take insulin, establish a regimen that replaces insulin at mealtimes and provides coverage throughout the day. Adjustment of your insulin doses should be based on your food intake and level of exercise.

Although these suggested guidelines are clear enough, many patients can't or won't comply. Why not? They may be unwilling to advance to insulin therapy because of the inconvenience or concern about injections. They may be unwilling to check their blood sugar on a regular basis, due to inconvenience or pain. Or they may not follow their nutritional or exercise plan consistently enough. Honestly, diabetes does require constant attention. It requires a change in eating and exercising. It requires keeping tabs on your blood sugar and maintaining healthy blood sugar levels. It may require taking medication. But as I will discuss in this book, there are newer strategies that you can use to overcome these barriers to care—and begin to live at your fullest capacity.

Understanding Diabetes

One of the basic things you'll want to grasp—and I hope your doctor has explained this to you—is an understanding of the natural history of diabetes; in other words, what type of diabetes do you have, how did it develop, and how will it progress? For background, diabetes is a group of metabolic diseases characterized by high blood sugar (glucose) levels, which result from defects in insulin secretion, action, or both.

There are two major forms of diabetes, referred to as type 1 and type 2 diabetes. Both types concern the relationship between blood glucose and insulin. Blood glucose refers to the amount of sugar measured in your blood. Your brain relies mostly on glucose for its nourishment; therefore, it must receive a fairly steady supply of glucose to function normally. Blood sugar normally rises after a meal and then returns to normal after several hours. Every moment of the day, blood sugar levels vary, with or without diabetes.

Insulin is a hormone produced by the pancreas, an elongated gland located behind your stomach. When you eat a meal, sugar enters the blood and causes your pancreas to release insulin. Insulin "opens the doors" of your cells so that glucose can be ushered inside and used for energy. As glucose enters the cells, your blood sugar level falls back to normal, and the release of insulin recedes until the next time you eat. Without adequate insulin, your cells cannot utilize glucose. Diabetes develops when insulin is not produced in sufficient amounts by the pancreas—a condition termed *insulin deficiency*—or cells don't respond to insulin properly—a condition called *insulin resistance*. In both situations, glucose is unable to enter cells readily and it starts increasing in the bloodstream—a condition called *hyperglycemia*, or high blood sugar. Over time, high blood sugar can damage organs such as the eyes, kidney, heart, and blood vessels.

There are important distinctions in the progression of each type of diabetes and their treatment. Once called juvenile-onset diabetes, type 1 diabetes is a disease in which the body attacks insulin-producing cells in the pancreas, the organ in the body that produces insulin. Children (or young adults) who develop this type of diabetes need insulin from the start of the disease in order to survive. However, type 2 diabetes, formerly called adult-onset diabetes, is by far the most common form of diabetes. Type 2 diabetes typically involves insulin resistance. However, insulin resistance does not cause diabetes. Fortunately, the knowledge and tools are here now to arrest the problems associated with both types of diabetes.

Type 1 Diabetes

Type 1 diabetes accounts for approximately 10 percent of all diabetes cases. It is considered an autoimmune disease. In type 1 diabetes, insulin-producing cells called *beta cells* in the pancreas are destroyed by the body's immune system. The body's immune system normally searches out and annihilates outside invaders such as viruses or bacteria. In a process that is not well understood, the body thinks that the beta cells are foreign and sets up an autoimmune response that ends up attacking those cells. Consequently, the ability to produce insulin is greatly reduced and people with type 1 diabetes must take insulin to survive. Without insulin, blood glucose rises. This oversupply of glucose, if left unchecked, can damage large and small blood vessels, doing serious damage to the body. Another consequence of no insulin is the production of harmful acids in the body. This results in ketoacidosis, a condition that if not treated aggressively can lead to death. Fortunately, doctors can now recognize this problem and catch the disease in its earlier stages; therefore, ketoacidosis is not as common.

Type 2 Diabetes

Type 2 diabetes accounts for approximately 90 percent of diagnosed cases and for almost all of those that go undiagnosed. It is generally preceded by a condition called prediabetes, which is marked by blood sugar levels that may be either normal or higher than normal but not high enough to be considered diabetes. Prediabetes goes by two other names: impaired glucose tolerance, and impaired fasting glucose. People diagnosed with prediabetes are usually insulin resistant, as well. It has been suggested that of all individuals who have prediabetes, up to 70 percent eventually develop diabetes. However, if you are diagnosed with prediabetes, you can take some simple steps to delay the progression to diabetes. It is never too early or too late to interrupt this disease process.

Although type 2 diabetes is preceded by prediabetes, it may not be diagnosed until complications appear. Once seen primarily in adults, type 2 diabetes has been rising steadily in children and teens, especially black, Hispanic, and Native American adolescents.

In type 2 diabetes, the body may produce insulin, though not enough of it to maintain blood sugar in the normal range for your body's needs. The body's tissues are insulin resistant as a result, and cells are less efficient at using insulin to process blood sugar. Insulin resistance is also associated with high levels of certain fats in the blood, high blood pressure, and obesity. In fact, most people who have this type of diabetes are overweight. Even if you do not have type 2 diabetes, obesity is a major risk factor for it. If you are overweight, you can control your condition by slimming down through diet and exercise. Even moderate weight loss can regulate blood sugar, reduce your risk of heart disease (a serious complication of diabetes), and can prevent the development of type 2 diabetes in those with prediabetes. Clearly, weight loss is a key therapeutic strategy if you have type 2 diabetes or are at risk of developing it.

Type 2 diabetes is a progressive disease. In the initial stages, you may be able to adequately control your blood glucose with diet and exercise only. Over time though, your pancreas will produce less and less insulin. This fact, combined with insulin resistance, makes it imperative that you add medical therapies, such as oral diabetes medications, to your diet and exercise programs, in order to keep your glucose levels in check. You may start off with one pill. Eventually, you may need two pills, and later, you may need insulin in addition to the pills. This is simply good medicine, and your ticket to a longer, more vigorous life. My entire approach to treating diabetes involves monitoring its progression and making sure my patients are controlling their blood sugar to halt that progression, even if it requires oral medication, insulin, or both.

Let me emphasize: just because you are on a pill does not mean you can abandon lifestyle measures like diet and exercise. *Everything works together to keep your blood sugar corralled.* Simply accept the fact that you may need the advanced therapy of medication and that the effects of the medication working with your lifestyle changes are controlling your blood sugar. Later in this book, I will discuss the various medications and which ones are right for you.

Gestational Diabetes

There is a third type of diabetes referred to as gestational diabetes. It develops during pregnancy, most often between twenty-four and twenty-eight weeks of gestation. With gestational diabetes, a woman experiences high levels of glucose when she is pregnant. This form of diabetes usually improves considerably when the pregnancy ends, with maintenance of normal blood sugar. Gestational diabetes must be diagnosed properly and treated promptly because it increases the risk of producing a larger than normal baby, and a large baby may have difficulty during delivery, or may be born by Cesarean section.

Fortunately, healthy behaviors, including good nutrition, exercise, and keeping your blood sugar within a normal range, can help prevent complications.

What May Be Missing from Your Current Treatment Plan

Despite everything we now know about treating all types of diabetes, more than one million new cases of the disease are diagnosed each year, according to the Centers for Disease Control and Prevention (CDC). Just what is wrong, and most important, why isn't current diabetes management working—and why might your treatment not be working optimally for you?

Reason #1: Prediabetes is not taken seriously.
By the time you are actually diagnosed with the disease, you may have had it for many years in the form of prediabetes. People with prediabetes may also have metabolic syndrome, characterized by excess weight in the abdominal area, high blood pressure, and abnormal blood lipids—all of which happen to be risk factors for heart disease. Fortunately, people with prediabetes and metabolic syndrome can take steps to prevent development of full-blown disease. But unfortunately, as a medical community, we are not aggressively advising prediabetics on how to take the necessary preventive measures, *even*

though *effective guidelines have been proven to reduce the progression in research studies.* Not surprisingly, the best approach to dealing with prediabetes is to change your lifestyle, by increasing physical activity and monitoring and reducing your food intake. This information comes primarily from the results of the Diabetes Prevention Program (DPP), a major clinical trial which showed that diet and exercise significantly reduced the chances that people with prediabetes will develop type 2 diabetes and, to a lesser degree, that the oral anti-diabetes drug metformin can reduce the risk as well.

Reason #2: There is a failure to meet recommended guidelines.
Patients with type 2 diabetes—who make up the vast majority of those with the disease—are not receiving management and treatment guidelines that could optimize their quality of life and significantly reduce their risk of developing complications, *even though these guidelines are known and proven.*

A case in point would be a woman I will call Louise, a forty-seven-year-old bank manager, who was recently diagnosed with type 2 diabetes. Both her mother and her older sister also have type 2 diabetes. Louise has been about thirty pounds overweight for the past fifteen years, and, until recently, rarely exercised. She has been taking blood pressure medication for several years. A year prior to her diagnosis, she had a fasting blood glucose level recorded at approximately 110 mg/dl, a value considered as impaired fasting glucose. In other words, she was prediabetic and would most likely progress to type 2 diabetes. Even so, it was never really stressed to Louise that she was at high risk for developing full-blown diabetes or what the complications might be. Although she was finally diagnosed with diabetes, her provider did not propose an aggressive plan that could greatly minimize her chances of complications.

"My doctor says I only have to check my blood glucose every three to four days, that I should exercise several times a week, and that I shouldn't eat sugar," says Louise. "Otherwise I don't need to make any big changes in my life."

Unfortunately, if Louise continues on this "program," and fails to reach suggested goals for blood sugar, blood pressure, and cholesterol levels, it is a good chance that the condition will progress and impose its own drastic changes in her life, changes she could avoid or at least greatly minimize if she were to follow sensible, proven guidelines. There may be too many people like Louise who have type 2 diabetes: living a lifestyle that promotes rather than seeks to eliminate or reduce the impact of diabetes.

Reason #3: Doctors aren't proactive enough about helping patients overcome common obstacles to compliance.

One major reason why this unfortunate situation continues is that as providers we have been led to believe that it is impossible for patients to change their lifestyle over a long-term period. Even research data supports the fact that patients are unsuccessful at maintaining lifestyle modifications over time. Why is this? First and foremost, although lifestyle strategies to help prevent or better manage diabetes can be easily incorporated into your daily life, these simple changes are not really stressed or routinely monitored in clinical practice. Secondly, we have at our disposal a vast array of newer drugs and devices, including newer glucose monitoring systems and insulin delivery systems that allow us to overcome many of the current barriers that exist for daily monitoring and insulin injection. However, many providers are not incorporating these into an intensive program to avoid the devastating consequences of the disease.

Take Action

Without a doubt, diabetes is serious, especially if left untreated, because it leads to dangerous health complications. About twenty-one million people in the United States have diabetes, with the majority having type 2 diabetes, and sadly, these numbers continue to rise. On a worldwide basis, it is expected that the cases of diabetes will double within the next twenty years, and in the United States alone, current estimates project almost a 60 percent increase. In certain ethnic populations, it is suggested that for every two individuals

---

ASK DR. CEFALU: WHY SHOULD I CARE ABOUT PREDIABETES OR DIABETES?

Diabetes is one of the leading causes of death in the United States, and prediabetes is on the rise. Having prediabetes increases your likelihood of developing the full-blown illness during your lifetime. Fortunately, diet and lifestyle changes can lower your odds and prevent the progression to diabetes. Even if you have neither condition, you may be impacted by someone who does—either a loved one, a family member, or close friend.

✳

born today, one will develop diabetes within their lifetime. The problem with this increase is that most people with diabetes will die of cardiovascular disease such as heart attack or stroke. As such, diabetes is considered one of the leading causes of death in this country.

You can fight back against diabetes using evidence from scientific studies practically applied to your life. If you are prediabetic, you'll learn how to reduce the risk of diabetes. If you have type 1 or type 2 diabetes, you'll learn how to significantly lower your chances of developing complications of the disease. This book gives you an overall program for taking charge of your diabetes and your life. It will work for you because it incorporates known successes from decades of research experience with diabetes and diabetic nutrition. The results of the research in these areas will be translated to an overall plan to successfully manage your diabetes. And it works because it is comprehensive.

My plan will start you off with a nutritional program you can easily follow. This is one of the biggest changes you'll make, since nutrition is the cornerstone of therapy. Very simply, nutrition to prevent or manage diabetes is all about healthy eating; it's the way all Americans should eat. You'll also learn about which nutritional supplements are worth taking—and those on which you may be wasting your money.

Another part of my plan involves ways to enhance your physical activity. I'm not talking about running marathons or doing hours of sweat-producing calisthenics. I'm talking about committing to at least thirty minutes of moderate-intensity physical activity a day. This might mean walking your children to the playground, or taking a stroll around the block during lunch or after dinner. That's it. Suffice it to say, small steps (literally) taken daily can be beneficial—and will do wonders to help prevent and manage diabetes.

For any diabetes plan to succeed, you have to stick with it—and there are now more ways than ever to stay on task. One of the most important is forming relationships with external sources to help support your diabetes management. Remember an important message of the DCCT study: frequent visits with a health-care team. While everyone doesn't have access to such a team, other support options are available and need to be utilized. My plan talks about those types of support and how to access them.

There is also a wide range of new and improved drugs and other treatments—including the potential of inhaled insulin and a class of newer drugs called incretins that control blood sugar and cause weight loss. I'll discuss with you how these medicines might fit into your overall treatment plan.

Essentially, therapy today means everything from diet and exercise to mixing and matching oral agents, to looking seriously at the addition of insulin when oral medications fail to adequately control blood sugar. These approaches improve quality of life—and save lives. In short, diabetes is something you do have to live with day in and day out, but you can still maintain an excellent quality of life.

With this book, I have undertaken the challenge of changing the course of diabetes. The latest critical information will be provided so that you can take the steps to prevent and manage the disease and its complications. Yes, diabetes is an epidemic, but I truly believe we have the knowledge and the resources to stem that tide—and in effect, stop diabetes.

ASK DR. CEFALU: IS THERE A CURE FOR DIABETES?

It depends on what you mean by "cure." Much progress has been made in the last few years toward prevention of diabetes, and I talk about them in this book. The most important thing is that you can prevent or delay the onset of complications or control the disease by living healthier. Moderate exercise helps your cells become more effective to utilize blood sugar and losing just 5 percent of your body weight with enhanced physical activity has been shown in research studies to significantly delay the progression to diabetes. This amount of weight loss if achieved once you have diabetes significantly improves glucose control. And if you're on diabetes medication, take it as prescribed and see your doctor regularly. These actions are vital until cures are available.

＊

Beware of Metabolic Syndrome and Prediabetes

DIABETES DOESN'T JUST APPEAR OUT OF the blue. It is a condition that develops stealthily, with its origins beginning many years before a diagnosis is made. Often, diabetes—namely type 2—stems from something called metabolic syndrome, or syndrome X—or from prediabetes. Both are conditions you don't want. If you have been diagnosed with either one, however, take heart. It is within your control to arrest metabolic syndrome and prediabetes, and by doing so, forestall diabetes.

Understanding Metabolic Syndrome

Metabolic syndrome describes a set of health risk factors that often occur together. These include excessive fat around the abdomen, blood fat disorders that lead to plaque buildup in arteries, insulin resistance, and high blood pressure, all of which weaken heart and metabolic health. Having these components of metabolic syndrome puts you at greater risk of developing heart disease and type 2 diabetes. This risk varies along a continuum; with each risk factor of the syndrome you have, your risk for heart disease goes up. Once type 2 diabetes emerges, the risk of heart disease increases even more.

There is resistance in the scientific community to using the term metabolic syndrome, since many of the components included in this condition independently predict heart disease. However, for the purposes of this book, I will use the term "metabolic syndrome" to define the clinical state present prior to development of diabetes and one that is associated with an increase in heart disease risk, or to be more specific, an increase in cardiometabolic risk.

Of the risk factors for metabolic syndrome, there are two in particular that serve as forecasters for future heart trouble: insulin resistance and abdominal obesity. Insulin resistance, as I discussed previously, occurs when your naturally produced insulin fails to deliver blood sugar into tissues. As such, it takes more and more insulin to keep blood glucose normal. Insulin resistance tends to occur when people gain weight.

Insulin resistance promotes changes in blood vessel walls that in turn begins the process leading to heart disease. Elevated insulin, a state technically called hyperinsulinemia, may also be associated with other heart disease risk factors that collectively promote greater cardiometabolic risk. For example:

- High triglycerides (fatty acids that circulate in the bloodstream);
- HDL ("good" cholesterol) that is too low;
- High LDL ("bad" cholesterol);
- Elevated blood clotting factors such as a compound called PAI-1 (plasminogen activator Inhibitor-1).

Abdominal fat, another factor pointing to metabolic syndrome, can also affect blood sugar metabolism. Why is this fat so hazardous? Abdominal fat cells work by readily expanding to accommodate more fuel. Essentially, the calories you eat over what you burn need to be stored somewhere, and that is the role of the fat cell (technically termed adipocyte). Thus, as the fat cells grow, more fuel is stored, widening your waist inch by inch.

In your abdominal region, there are essentially two types of fat tissue. The fat that you can squeeze at your waist between your fingers is called subcutaneous fat. In addition, there is a deep fat, layered among internal organs, such as the intestines, to cushion and protect them, and this is termed visceral fat or intra-abdominal fat. This fat may be metabolically more active than subcutaneous fat, meaning that it easily releases fatty acids into the bloodstream. These fat molecules released from the visceral fat head directly to the liver and into your circulation. This makes muscle cells inefficient at using your body's insulin, and insulin resistance develops. Insulin resistance is associated with high blood pressure, low HDL ("good" cholesterol), and high triglycerides (unhealthy blood fats)—all the conditions that are present in metabolic syndrome.

In a way, metabolic syndrome gives doctors a glimpse into a patient's future. We evaluate this syndrome in our patients because it tells us whether they're at greater risk for heart disease and diabetes, or not. When we know that the risk of either disease, or both, is increased in someone, we initiate treatment to avert it. This is called primary prevention, and it focuses on preventing the development of the disease. Once someone has heart disease, we try to prevent stroke or heart attack, and this is referred to as secondary prevention.

Do You Have Metabolic Syndrome?

You may wonder: what does all this mean to me? Is my own health at risk? How do I know if I have metabolic syndrome?

According to the National Cholesterol Education Panel, if you have at least three of the following characteristics, you're classified as having metabolic syndrome:

- Abdominal obesity (a waist size greater than 40 inches for men, and 35 inches for women).
- Triglyceride levels of 150 mg/dl or higher.
- HDL ("good" cholesterol) of less than 40 mg/dl in men and 50 mg/dl in women.
- Blood pressure of 130/85 mm Hg or higher.
- Fasting blood sugar of 110 (100*) mg/dl or more.

Clearly, metabolic syndrome presents a risk to your health. A study published in 2002 in the *Journal of the American Medical Association* showed just

---

* In 2003, the American Diabetes Association recommended lowering the limit for impaired fasting glucose from 110 mg/dl to 100 mg/dl.

how serious this risk is. Between 1984 and 1998, researchers at the University of Kuopio in Finland followed each of 1,209 Finnish men for an average of more than 11 years. All volunteers were initially between forty-two and sixty years old and free of heart disease, diabetes, and cancer. From tests at the beginning of the study, the researchers identified which men met criteria of the metabolic syndrome. Essentially, they needed to have three of the risk factors identified above. Participants who began the study with metabolic syndrome were between 2.9 and 4.2 times as likely to die of heart disease as were those without it.

In a decade-long Finnish study published in the *European Heart Journal*, the same researchers found that men with waist-to-hip ratios of 0.91 or greater nearly tripled their risk of heart disease. (The measure is calculated by dividing your waist circumference by the circumference at your hips.)

As you might imagine, it is very important to know your numbers: your cholesterol levels, blood pressure, blood sugar, and triglyceride levels (blood fats). Blood tests can determine whether you have high cholesterol or high triglyceride levels, and these are typically performed as a part of a routine physical examination. Usually, you'll have what is called a fasting test because you are not supposed to eat for eight to twelve hours before having your blood drawn. Your blood sugar is typically measured through one of two tests:

- *A fasting blood glucose test.* This test is the most recommended test and is the easiest to perform. After an eight-hour overnight fast, your blood is drawn and your blood sugar level measured to see whether it is within a normal range. If it is greater than 100 mg/dl but less than 125 mg/dl, you may have impaired fasting glucose.
- *Oral glucose tolerance test (OGTT).* This test is less frequently performed because of the time involved and because of the repeated blood draws. However, your doctor may elect to do this test if other tests, including the fasting blood level, is abnormal. This test measures blood glucose levels several times: once after fasting (for eight to sixteen hours) and again after one, two, or three hours after drinking liquid glucose. With the OGTT, normal blood glucose level two hours after the drink would be below 140 mg/dl; an elevated fasting blood glucose level < 126 mg/dl

and a two-hour value in the range of 140 to 199 mg/dl would be abnormal and considered as impaired glucose tolerance. Having impaired glucose tolerance indicates prediabetes, and a markedly increased chance of progressing to diabetes.

Based on looking at your test results, your physician can diagnose whether you have metabolic syndrome. However, it is a good idea to be alert to the presence of risk factors so you can bring them to your doctor's attention, as well as stay on top of them in order to note trends. One important factor not measured in these tests is a family history of heart disease. If you have family members with heart disease and if components of metabolic syndrome are present, your physician may have to be more aggressive in his recommendations. Here is a work sheet you can use to figure your risk:

Metabolic Syndrome Work Sheet

What to Measure	My Numbers	What My Results Mean
* My waist circumference:		A waist size greater than 40 inches for men, and 35 inches for women, is a risk factor for metabolic syndrome.
Triglycerides:		A value above 150 is a risk factor.
HDL cholesterol:		A value of less than 40 in men and less than 50 in women is a risk factor.
Blood pressure:		A reading of 130/85 or greater is a risk factor for metabolic syndrome.
Fasting blood glucose:		If your fasting blood glucose is 100 or above, this is a risk factor.
Number of risk factors I have:		Any of three of five risk factors constitutes the presence of metabolic syndrome.

* Waist circumference is a convenient way of measuring abdominal fat. Use a tape measure to find your waist circumference. To measure your waist accurately, place a tape measure around your bare abdomen just above your hip bone. Be sure that the tape is snug, but does not compress your skin, and is parallel to the floor. Relax, exhale, and measure your waist.

How Is Metabolic Syndrome Treated?

Metabolic syndrome can be easily treated with lifestyle modifications, including proper diet and moderate physical activity. Because abnormalities in blood vessels may ultimately lead to problems with heart disease years down the road, it is quite possible that you will need prescription medications to help control your blood lipids and blood pressure. In addition, if your blood glucose is abnormal, your physician may elect to provide you with medication to control it too.

Not long ago, I worked with a teacher at a local high school, Richard, age fifty-four. He confessed to me that he had a very inactive lifestyle and he ate a lot of fast food. "I get to work early and have a lot of paperwork in the afternoon. I generally have coffee and a muffin on the way to work, and whatever fast-food sandwich I can grab at lunch. Yep, French fries are included," he admitted. "I just don't have a lot of time."

Fitting in exercise was tough for him. "After school, I check up on my e-mail and surf the Internet. I'm generally too tired to do any activity," he told me.

When we examined him, Richard had a blood pressure of 150/90 (very high), a fasting glucose of 103 mg/dl, a BMI of 33, and a triglyceride level of 350 mg/dl (very high). He was not diabetic yet, but diabetes was knocking on the door. His grouping of symptoms pointed to metabolic syndrome.

We sent Richard to our registered dietitian who instructed him on some very simple steps to take charge of his life. He began to make time for a healthier breakfast of oatmeal or whole-grain cereal, and healthy sandwiches or salads for lunch. He started a simple walking program with some of his other faculty at school and bought a pedometer to measure his steps. I also put him on blood pressure medication.

"I have now lost thirty pounds. I walk three miles four days a week. My glucose is 95 mg/dl, my triglycerides are 160 mg/dl, and I have more energy today than I have had for the past twenty years," he proudly reported. Essentially, Richard got his metabolic syndrome under control, and delayed progression to serious illness.

As with Richard's case, the goal of treatment is to reduce the known risk factors for heart disease and diabetes. Treatment involves:

Weight control. This is your first priority if you are overweight and have excessive abdominal fat. Losing weight is very effective in reducing all risk factors for heart disease and remains as a cornerstone of treatment, even when medications are added. Weight loss occurs when your energy expenditure (calories burned during daily activities) is greater over time than your energy intake (calories consumed). The caloric amount for you to lose weight needs to be balanced by the calories you require for your daily activities. For example, if you are in the construction business and have a very active job, naturally you'll require more calories on a daily basis (but less than you were eating prior to a diet) than someone who has a desk job and is inactive. The number of calories you require daily for weight loss varies, based on your current level of physical activity, gender, and size. You can arrive at the right calorie formula by consulting with a dietitian.

As to how much weight to lose, most would agree that you should aim to reduce weight by 5 to 10 percent. For example, if you are a very active male, with a body weight of two hundred fifty pounds, and your doctor tells you that you have developed impaired fasting glucose, a goal for weight loss for you would be calculated by multiplying 250 pounds times .05 and 250 pounds times .1. Essentially, your ideal range of weight loss as a preventive strategy would be 12.5 pounds (5 percent weight loss) to 25 pounds (10 percent weight loss).

In addition to total calories, choose fats wisely, too. Opt for monounsaturated and polyunsaturated (fish, nuts, canola and olive oils) over the saturated varieties (red meat, potato chips, whole-milk dairy products, coconut and palm oils). Use only small amounts of butter or use a margarine that has no transfatty acids, and buy leaner cuts of meat.

Physical activity. Along with these nutrition recommendations, try to engage in moderate-intensity physical activity thirty minutes a day, most days of the week, to help you shed pounds. For preventing and treating metabolic syndrome, exercise is especially effective because it decreases insulin resistance, helps lower blood pressure, and fights other factors related to heart disease, such as obesity. If you can increase your exercise time to sixty minutes a day, all the better. You can break your exercise up into multiple short (ten to fifteen minutes) bouts of activity too. However, before you embark on any exercise program, and particularly if you haven't exercised for a while and have had the risk factors mentioned, *it will be important to have your physician evaluate you first to ensure there are no underlying medical or heart problems that would complicate an exercise program.* Your physician may elect to do specific screening tests that include a way to "image" or look at the function of your heart. This is very important as you may have gone undiagnosed for many years and may indeed have problems with your heart even though you don't have symptoms.

Normalize your blood pressure. The goal of blood pressure management if you have diabetes is to reduce blood pressure to less than 130/80. Consider purchasing a home blood pressure monitoring device. Measure and record your blood pressure, and bring this information to your doctor during each office visit. Dietary change can help, particularly with the regulation of your salt and sodium intake, and is important in reaching your treatment goal.

Smoking cessation. If you are a smoker, enrolling in a smoking-cessation program is essential. There is no question that active smoking confers a high risk for heart disease.

The earlier you take action, the better. By committing yourself to certain lifestyle changes, the greater your potential to prevent progression to diabetes and heart disease.

Metabolic Syndrome and Prediabetes

"Prediabetes" means having early metabolic abnormalities that precede the development of type 2 diabetes. It includes having either impaired fasting glucose or impaired glucose tolerance. A fasting glucose ranging between 100 and 125 mg/dl is considered as impaired fasting glucose. A two-hour plasma glucose value greater than 140 mg/dl but less than 200 mg/dl is termed impaired glucose tolerance. Another way to define prediabetes is higher-than-normal blood sugar, although not high enough to be called diabetes. With prediabetes, you also have more of a risk for developing heart disease and other associated complications. Approximately 26 percent of U.S. adults are estimated to have prediabetes, or impaired fasting glucose. Add that to the number of people with diabetes, and you'll find that seventy-three million Americans have prediabetes or diabetes.

Fortunately, we do know that lifestyle changes are effective in treating prediabetes. For example, if you lose 5 to 7 percent of your body weight—which is about twelve to eighteen pounds for someone who weighs two hundred fifty pounds—by making modest changes in your diet and level of physical activity, you stand a good chance of arresting the progression of prediabetes to diabetes.

Could You Have Prediabetes and Not Know It?

How do you know if you have prediabetes? Unfortunately, prediabetes can develop without any discernable signs or symptoms, and may progress to type 2 diabetes without major symptoms initially. The classic symptoms of diabetes include frequent urination and excessive thirst, lack of energy, weight loss, blurred vision, or a feeling of being tired most of the time for no apparent reason. Sometimes, the symptoms are there, but they appear so gradually that they aren't recognized.

Prediabetes can be detected through simple blood tests such as obtaining a fasting blood glucose test. With the skyrocketing epidemic in prediabetes and diabetes, knowing your blood sugar level is as important as knowing your cholesterol levels. The American Diabetes Association has developed the following recommendations for testing for prediabetes:

- If you are over the age of forty-five, you should be tested during a routine medical office visit. If the screening test is normal, it should be repeated once every three years.
- Testing should be considered at a younger age or be carried out more frequently in individuals who are overweight and have additional risk factors such as:
  - A sedentary lifestyle;
  - Having a first-degree relative with diabetes;
  - Being a member of a high-risk ethnic population (such as African-American, Latino, Native American, Asian American, Pacific Islander);
  - Having a history of gestational diabetes or giving birth to a baby weighing more than nine pounds;
  - Having high blood pressure equal to or greater than 140/90;

- A low level of HDL ("good" cholesterol) (less than 35 mg/dl);
- High triglycerides (greater than 250 mg/dl);
- Having a history of vascular disease;
- Testing positive for impaired glucose tolerance or impaired fasting glucose on a previous test.

The Science Behind Stopping Prediabetes

Major proof that the progression of prediabetes to diabetes comes from several landmark studies. One is called the Diabetes Prevention Program (DPP), which was sponsored by the National Institutes of Health. In this study, more than three thousand overweight men and women from twenty-seven clinical centers around the country were randomly split into different treatment groups. The first group, called the lifestyle intervention group, received intensive training in diet, exercise, and behavior modification. They ate less fat and fewer calories and exercised for a total of one hundred fifty minutes a week.

The second group took 850 milligrams of metformin (Glucophage) twice a day to lower their blood sugar. The third group received placebo pills instead of metformin. The metformin and placebo groups also received information on diet and exercise, but no intensive counseling efforts. A fourth group was treated with the drug troglitazone (Rezulin), but this part of the study was discontinued after researchers discovered that troglitazone can cause serious liver damage. Rezulin is no longer on the U.S. market.

All of the participants had impaired glucose tolerance, a well-recognized risk factor for the development of type 2 diabetes. In addition, 45 percent of the participants were from minority groups—African-American, Hispanic American/Latino, Asian American or Pacific Islander, or Native American—known to be at considerable risk of developing diabetes.

The results were so impressive that the researchers stopped the trial a year earlier than was planned. For example:

Participants in the lifestyle intervention group—those receiving intensive counseling on effective diet, exercise, and behavior modification—reduced their risk of developing diabetes by 58 percent. This finding was true across all participating ethnic groups and for both men and women. Lifestyle changes worked particularly well for participants aged sixty and older, reducing their risk by 71 percent. The researchers think that weight loss—achieved through better eating habits and exercise—reduces the risk of diabetes by improving the ability of the body to use insulin and process glucose.

Those people taking metformin reduced their risk of developing diabetes by 31 percent. Metformin was effective for both men and women, but it was least effective in people aged forty-five and older. Metformin worked best for people twenty-five to forty-four years old and in those at least sixty pounds overweight, suggesting that the drug may have merit in postponing the onset of diabetes.

These results were powerful because they showed that losing a little weight and enhancing physical activity was enough to make a difference. It's the small lifestyle changes that really add up. You'll learn how to make the very same changes made by the participants in the DPP.

The second study I want to tell you about is called the Finnish Diabetes Prevention Study. In this study, 522 overweight people, aged forty to sixty-five years, with impaired glucose tolerance (prediabetes) were randomized into two groups: either an intensive lifestyle intervention or a control group, and were followed for 3.2 years. The lifestyle intervention group followed a five-point plan: get half an hour of exercise daily; lose 5 percent of your total weight; reduce your fat intake to 30 percent of total calories; cut your saturated fat intake to less than 10 percent of total calories; and eat more fiber (more fruits, veggies, and whole grains). The control group was given general information on diet and exercise, but without individualized programs.

The results of this study closely mirrored the findings in the DPP study: those in the lifestyle intervention group who took four of those five steps significantly prevented the progression to diabetes. What this tells us is that the right lifestyle changes can prevent type 2 diabetes.

There is even more reason for optimism that type 2 diabetes can be prevented. In a study called the Troglitazone in Prevention of Diabetes (TRIPOD) study, 235 Hispanic women with a history of gestational diabetes (which is a strong risk factor for the development of type 2 diabetes) were randomized to receive either troglitazone (Rezulin), before it was removed from the U.S. market, or a placebo. Troglitazone is a drug from a class of compounds called thiazolidinediones that improve the body's efficiency to insulin (insulin sensitizers). There is a whole chapter devoted to discussing these and other drugs for diabetes.

After a follow-up of thirty months, the women who received troglitazone had a 56 percent reduction in the development of diabetes. Women who had received troglitizone before its removal from the market still had a beneficial effect during the eight months of the study that took place after the drug was stopped. This suggests that improving insulin resistance through oral diabetes medications was also effective for delaying the progression to diabetes.

A more definitive study was recently completed with newer diabetes drugs. This study, called the DREAM Trial (the Diabetes Reduction Assessment with Ramipril and Rosiglitazone Medication), showed that 8 milligrams of rosi-glitazone (Avandia) administered daily for three years significantly reduced the progression to type 2 diabetes and reverted blood sugar to normal among a large proportion of adults with impaired fasting glucose (IFG), impaired glucose tolerance (IGT), or both. IFG and IGT are hallmarks of prediabetes. Unfortunately, it is noted that with the use of the drugs that increased insulin sensitivity—in this case, rosiglitazone—there was also a significant increase in congestive heart failure. So, the bottom line is there were benefits to this particular drug to prevent diabetes, but also risk involved.

What are the implications to you of these studies? First and foremost, I believe that if the early steps to developing diabetes are recognized and a program put in place, there is a great chance that progression to diabetes can be reduced dramatically. This is positive, promising news. Second, taken to-gether, the DPP and the Finnish study suggest that type 2 diabetes can be de-layed or prevented with a safe, inexpensive therapy, such as losing weight, changing dietary habits, and exercising. The plan I've outlined for you in this book, from nutrition to exercise to medication, is based on this research, and you'll discover how to apply it easily to your life.

If you learn that you have prediabetes, you have the opportunity to prevent or substantially delay the development of full-blown diabetes. It does take a serious commitment to certain lifestyle changes, but these changes are entirely doable—and that's powerfully positive news.

The Good and Bad News about Complications

TRUE OR FALSE? YOU CAN'T ESCAPE THE complications of diabetes. Happily, the correct answer is false. In just the past ten years, we have learned that not only can progression to diabetes be prevented, but also that its devastating complications can be halted. We know through major studies that making changes in diet and exercise and improving glucose control forestalls complications. We now have better techniques to help patients achieve glucose control. But the brutal reality is that if left unchecked, diabetes leads to damage to your vital organs.

This damage can be far ranging, from your eyes to your feet, and is caused by uncontrolled blood sugar that persists over time. Diabetes can damage cells in the retina and lens of your eyes. It can also hurt the filtration system of the kidneys and can kill nerves. With deadened nerves, your feet feel numb, making them injury prone. Because blood flow slows down, wounds heal more slowly, and infections can get out of hand. Diabetes remains one of the leading causes of blindness, kidney failure, amputations, and heart disease. As many as twenty-four thousand diabetics in the United States become blind each year, more than one hundred thousand require dialysis or kidney transplantation, and eighty-two thousand need to have a toe, foot, or leg amputated. The combination of nerve and circulatory damage causes many diabetic men to become impotent. Large blood vessels are damaged too, creating the most common lethal complications of diabetes such as heart attack and stroke.

Why is diabetes so damaging? Chronically high levels of blood sugar cause glucose to attach, or become glycated to oxygen-carrying hemoglobin in red blood cells and to other proteins in your body. The process of glycation—the binding of glucose to hemoglobin or other substances—is damaging to blood vessels over time. Once hemoglobin becomes glycated, it stays that way throughout the life span of the red blood cell, which is about two to three months. The more glucose you have in your blood, the more hemoglobin will become glycated. The A1c test can thus tell your doctor how well your glucose has been controlled over the past three months.

Fortunately, there is more good news than bad in the treatment of diabetes and its complications: the future for anyone with diabetes and its complications has never been brighter. You are not as helpless against the ravages of diabetes as we once thought, especially if the disease is detected at its very earliest stages. Tight control of glucose, along with changes in lifestyle and diet and use of effective medications can, in the vast majority of cases, make a huge difference. Should complications develop, the prognosis is not unrelentingly grim either. Laser surgery can save eyesight. Aggressive medical therapy for heart problems is effective. And medications to improve abnormalities in the kidneys are available.

One of the main purposes of this book is to translate some of the important—and amazing—science proving that we can prevent progression to diabetes, control diabetes once you have it, and manage its complications effectively. I want to elaborate on a study I mentioned earlier: the United Kingdom Prospective Diabetes Study (UKPDS), which began in 1977 at Oxford University. It followed more than five thousand people with type 2 diabetes. The goal of the study was to understand the best way to manage the disease and to prevent or delay its serious complications. The average age of the participants was fifty-three years old, and they were divided into groups receiving intensive or medical treatment, and conventional treatment, which consisted of lifestyle interventions primarily.

Now the remarkable news: in 1998 when the findings were published, the researchers reported that intensively controlling glucose significantly reduced kidney damage, eye damage, and possibly, nerve damage. Specifically, better blood glucose control reduced the risk of major diabetic eye disease by a quarter, and early kidney damage by a third. In the many people with high blood pressure, better blood pressure control reduced the risk of death from long-term complications of diabetes by a third, strokes by more than a third, and serious deterioration of vision by more than a third.

The bottom line? Diabetic complications are not inevitable. They can be prevented in many cases, while in others their impact can be significantly reduced. So if the threat of diabetic complications has you worried—and well it should—you have control over the development and progression. In controlling the complications, you'll enjoy a better quality of life.

Lifesaving Medical Care

In early stages, complications of diabetes are often silent, but they can creep up on you and put your life at risk—which is why you need regular physical examinations and laboratory tests as a part of your ongoing diabetes care. As doctors, we use tests to detect complications, gauge their progress, and prescribe corrective action to effectively treat or halt the progression of the problem.

As part of initiating ongoing care, your doctor will take a detailed medical history that looks for signs of complications, including eye, kidney, nerve, bladder, gastrointestinal, and heart problems. You'll also cover lifestyle issues such as diet, exercise, smoking, family history, medications you're taking, prior or current infections, and really anything that might influence your diabetes management. Additionally, your doctor will:

- Check your blood pressure.
- Look in your eyes for signs of eye disease.
- Touch your neck to feel your thyroid.
- Listen to your heart and lungs.

- Take your pulse.
- Test your reflexes, check your limbs for signs of nerve damage.

You'll undergo laboratory tests to see how well you're controlling your blood sugar and controlling other risk factors. Your age, complications, and symptoms dictate which other laboratory tests your doctor does. The general tests you'll have include:

- *Fasting Plasma Glucose.* Mentioned earlier, this test checks your blood for evidence of high blood sugar. After you have fasted overnight for at least eight hours, a blood sample is drawn and analyzed. After fasting, normal blood sugar levels are less than 100 mg/dl. If blood sugar exceeds 126 mg/dl, this is considered in the diabetic range.
- *Hemoglobin A1c test.* Also known as the glycated hemoglobin, or A1c, test, this blood test checks your average blood sugar level over two to three months. As I described earlier, glucose in the blood sticks to hemoglobin, a protein in red blood cells that transports oxygen, forming glycated hemoglobin. Because red blood cells circulate in the body for several months, levels of glycated hemoglobin are a good marker for how well you've been controlling your glucose levels for the past three months. For patients not meeting their blood sugar goals, a doctor will probably do this test quarterly. Normal A1c is generally considered approximately 6 percent or less, depending on the lab. The American Diabetes Association suggests a value no higher than 7 percent, but the lower the value the better.
- *Thyroid function test(s) when indicated.* If your doctor suspects a thyroid problem, thyroid function tests will be ordered, since diabetic patients have a higher prevalence of thyroid disorders compared with the general population. These tests check how well your thyroid gland is working. The thyroid gland makes hormones that regulate your metabolism. An overactive thyroid may cause weight loss and heart palpitations, while an underactive thyroid can raise your bad cholesterol levels.
- *Serum creatinine.* Creatinine is a waste product in your blood that comes from muscle activity. It is normally removed from your blood by your kidneys, but when kidney function slows down, the creatinine level rises. A normal value is generally less than 1.2 mg/dl for males and

1.1 mg/dl for females. Your doctor may use the results of your serum creatinine test to calculate your glomerular filtration rate (GFR). Your GFR tells how much kidney function you have. If your GFR falls below 30, you may need to see a kidney disease specialist (called a nephrologist). Your kidney doctor will speak to you about treatments for kidney failure like dialysis or kidney transplant.

- **Urinalysis.** This test is performed to check for protein in your urine. If protein is present (a condition called proteinuria), your doctor will order additional testing to help determine appropriate treatment. If protein is not present, a test will be done to see whether you have very small amounts of a specific protein called albumin in your urine (a condition called microalbuminuria), which cannot be detected with a routine urinalysis. Protein in the urine can be a sign of kidney damage.

- **Urine culture.** This test detects and identifies bacteria or fungi that may be causing a urinary tract infection (UTI). The type of organisms causing the infection is identified with a microscope or by chemical tests. Generally, this test may only be done if you are known to have an infection in the urine.

- **Fasting lipid profile.** This is a fasting blood test that measures your blood lipids: LDL ("bad" cholesterol), HDL ("good" cholesterol), total cholesterol, and triglycerides. High cholesterol and triglycerides can increase your risk for developing cardiovascular complications associated with diabetes, so it is important to know whether your cholesterol and triglyceride levels are healthy or need treatment. The chart below provides information on blood fats values and what they mean. However, there is data suggesting that if you are either nondiabetic or diabetic and have heart disease with multiple risk factors, the goal of an LDL of 100 mg/dl may still be too high. In this regard, LDL levels well below 70 may be the goal for you. Thus, the level of LDL suggested for your condition will need to be discussed with your physician based on the other risk factors you have.

- **Electrocardiogram.** This test checks your heart function. It is usually done even if you have not had a heart attack or do not have heart disease, because people with diabetes are at such a high risk for heart disease.

- **An exercise stress test.** This test provides information about how your heart responds to exertion. It usually involves walking on a treadmill at

Total Cholesterol	Interpretation
Less than 200	Desirable
200–239	Borderline High
240 and above	High
LDL Cholesterol Levels	
Less than 100 mg/dl	Optimal
100–129 mg/dl	Near Optimal/Above Optimal
130 and above	Elevated
HDL Cholesterol	
Less than 40 mg/dl	Low
Greater than 60 mg/dl	High (which is optimal)
Triglycerides	
Less than 150 mg/dl	Normal
150–199 mg/dl	Borderline High
200–499 mg/dl	High
500 mg/dl or higher	Very High

increasing levels of difficulty, while your electrocardiogram, heart rate, and blood pressure are monitored. This test determines if there is adequate blood flow to your heart during increasing levels of activity, identifies the presence of abnormal heart rhythm, and detects the likelihood of heart disease. It is a good test to have prior to beginning an exercise program. Generally this test may be done at the same time your doctor also does an imaging study, which when coupled with the stress test may be a more sensitive test to determine if a heart problem exists.

Other Tests

Although not routinely done, your doctor may choose to do other tests depending on your condition and risk factors. One of these tests may be a C-reactive protein (CRP) test. This is a blood test that measures the concentration of a protein in serum that indicates inflammation, which is associated with heart disease and other diseases. A normal CRP value varies from lab to lab. Treating conditions such as abnormal lipids or obesity will reduce an elevated level.

An Overview of the Major Complications of Diabetes

Often, the first clue that you have diabetes is that you develop complications. Doctors talk about microvascular complications, those affecting small blood vessels, and macrovascular complications, those affecting large blood vessels such as the arteries. What follows is a closer look at some of the major complications of diabetes, and how to treat them.

Small Vessel ("Microvascular") Complications

RETINOPATHY

Diabetic retinopathy, damage in the small blood vessels of the retina, is the most frequent cause of blindness among adults between the ages of twenty and seventy-four years. Between twelve thousand and twenty-four thousand new cases of blindness due to retinopathy occur each year. Nearly all patients with type 1 diabetes have some degree of retinopathy after twenty years, as do more than 60 percent of those with type 2 diabetes. It is the most common eye disease related to diabetes and is twice as likely as cataracts and glaucoma to afflict people with diabetes—so you want to prevent it at all costs.

Over time, diabetes affects the circulatory system of the retina, which is the light-sensitive tissue at the back of the eye. In some people with diabetes, the blood vessels in the retina are observed to swell and leak fluid. In others, it is noted that abnormal new blood vessels grow on the surface of the retina. If you have diabetic retinopathy, you may not notice changes to your vision at first. But over time, the retinopathy can get worse and cause vision loss. Diabetic retinopathy usually affects both eyes.

Even so, its progression can be arrested with tighter blood sugar control. A case in point is Polly, age fifty-six, who has had type 1 diabetes for twenty-six years but has never had adequate control of her disease. Her A1c levels, for example, have ranged from around 7.8 to 9.5 percent over the years, indicating poor control. Her doctor had her on two injections of a mixture of a short- and long-acting insulin twice daily. Polly was never interested in advancing to a more intensive insulin regimen because of the "hassle."

"I was a busy person and really didn't have time to inject myself three or four times a day. I was also worried about the possibility of low blood sugar with that many injections." Employed as a real estate agent, Polly had erratic eating habits and a hectic schedule. She told me, "I could not afford to have the low blood sugar feeling when I was with a client."

With her diabetes going uncontrolled for so long, Polly's vision began to go, and it happened suddenly and without warning. When evaluated by her ophthalmologist, she was told she had a "vitreous hemorrhage."

"I was in total shock! One day I could see well, the next I was seeing the world through badly unfocused glasses!"

Polly had a procedure called vitrectomy (see page 43) and has since had multiple laser treatments on her eyes to prevent further bleeding. In consultation with her endocrinologist, she is now on an insulin pump as a way to deliver intensive insulin therapy—which works better for her than having to do injections. She now checks her blood glucoses four times a day, and her A1c was last recorded at 6.8 percent.

"I was told that I can never turn back the clock and have my vision as it was years ago," Polly admits. "But I am now comforted by the knowledge that if I control my blood sugar, I can stop further damage to my eyes."

The National Eye Institute of the National Institutes of Health has provided information on four stages of retinopathy, and more information is available from its Web site. These stages consist of:

1. **Mild nonproliferative retinopathy.** This is considered the earliest stage, and at this stage, there are microaneurysms, small areas of balloonlike swelling in the retina's tiny blood vessels.
2. **Moderate nonproliferative retinopathy.** As this stage of retinopathy, some blood vessels that nourish the retina are blocked.
3. **Severe nonproliferative retinopathy.** As retinopathy progresses, many more blood vessels are blocked. This deprives several areas of the retina with their blood supply. Signals from these areas of the retina are sent to the body to grow new blood vessels for nourishment.

4. **Proliferative retinopathy.** At this advanced stage, the signals sent by the retina for nourishment trigger the growth of new blood vessels. Unfortunately, these new blood vessels are abnormal and fragile. They grow along the retina and along the surface of the clear, vitreous gel that fills the inside of the eye. The problem with this new growth of blood vessels is that they may leak blood because they have thin, fragile walls. If they leak blood, this is associated with the severe vision loss and blindness.

Screening for Retinopathy If you are diagnosed with either type 1 or type 2 diabetes, you should follow specific recommendations for screening. Having routine eye exams, along with tight control of glucose, can go a long way to toward preventing retinopathy, or delaying its progression. Here are specific screening guidelines as suggested by the American Diabetes Association:

- If you are an adult or an adolescent with type 1 diabetes, have an initial dilated and comprehensive eye examination by an ophthalmologist or optometrist within three to five years after the onset of your diabetes.
- If you have type 2 diabetes, have an initial dilated and comprehensive eye examination by an ophthalmologist or optometrist shortly after the diagnosis of your diabetes.
- If you have type 1 or type 2 diabetes, after the initial recommended evaluation, you should have annual examinations by an ophthalmologist or optometrist. If your eye exam is normal, you may need less frequent exams (every two to three years), but that should be determined by the eye specialist. But if retinopathy is progressing, you'll require more frequent eye exams.
- If you are a woman who is planning a pregnancy or who has become pregnant, you should have a comprehensive eye examination and should be counseled on the risk of development and/or progression of diabetic retinopathy. Your eye examination should occur in the first trimester with close follow-up throughout pregnancy and for one year after you have your baby. This guideline does not apply if you develop gestational diabetes because you are not at increased risk for diabetic retinopathy.

Preventing Retinopathy Like most complications of type 1 and type 2 diabetes, retinopathy is associated with poor glucose control. However, you can reduce the risk of developing it or slow its progression by keeping your blood sugar within normal limits. (For detailed information on controlling your blood sugar, see Chapter 8.)

Treating Retinopathy If diagnosed with retinopathy, you have treatment options, depending on the severity of the condition, in order to prevent the loss of your vision. With mild nonproliferative retinopathy, you may not require treatment right away, although your eye doctor should closely monitor your eyes, and your retina in particular.

Severe retinopathy and proliferative retinopathy usually require more aggressive intervention, however. One of the main interventions for retinopathy is laser photocoagulation. The goal of photocoagulation is to stop the leakage of blood and fluid in the retina and thus slow the progression of diabetic retinopathy and vision loss. With this procedure, a high-energy laser beam is used to help seal any leaks in areas of the retina with abnormal blood vessels. The procedure takes place in your ophthalmologist's office on an outpatient basis, usually over several visits. Two large-scale National Institutes of Health–sponsored trials, the Diabetic Retinopathy Study (DRS) and the Early Treatment Diabetes Retinopathy Study (ETDRS), provided strong support for the effectiveness of photocoagulation surgery.

During the early stages of diabetic retinopathy, no treatment may be needed. However, it is recommended that to prevent progression of diabetic retinopathy, people with diabetes should have their levels of blood sugar, blood pressure, and blood cholesterol adequately controlled.

If you have proliferative retinopathy, your doctor may suggest laser surgery. Scatter laser treatment is done to shrink the abnormal blood vessels. To do this procedure, your doctor places one thousand to two thousand laser burns in the areas of the retina away from the macula, causing the abnormal blood vessels to shrink. It may take two or more sessions to complete treatment. This procedure can save the rest of your sight. This procedure works better before the fragile, new blood vessels have started to bleed. That is why it is important to have regular, comprehensive screening visits for eye problems.

If the bleeding is excessive, you may need a surgical procedure called a vitrectomy. For a vitrectomy, your surgeon uses delicate instruments to treat the blood-filled vitreous. A vitreous cutter cuts the tissue and removes it, piece by piece, from your eye, in order to establish clear vision. The tissue that is removed is replaced with a balanced salt solution to maintain the normal shape and pressure of the eye.

NEPHROPATHY

Diabetic nephropathy is a kidney disease that occurs as a result of diabetes and is the leading cause of kidney failure for individuals who ultimately need dialysis. In people who have had diabetes for many years, the filtering system in the kidneys becomes severely compromised and unable to filter out toxins. This is more likely to occur if your blood sugar has been poorly controlled over many years.

Screening for Nephropathy One of the first detectable signs of diabetic nephropathy is microalbuminuria, the leakage of small amounts of a specific blood protein, called albumin, from the blood into the urine. Microalbuminuria is one of the most important predictors for the risk of progressing to kidney disease in patients with diabetes. It has thus become a very crucial measure in the care of patients. If you have had type 1 diabetes for five years or more, you should be screened on a yearly basis for microalbuminuria. If you have type 2 diabetes, you should be screened, beginning at diagnosis, and on a yearly basis thereafter.

Diabetic nephropathy is not inevitable after onset of microalbuminuria, and aggressive therapy is indicated to prevent further kidney damage. Case in point: In a six-year study published in the *New England Journal of Medicine*, researchers found that controlling blood sugar, blood pressure, and cholesterol could reduce microalbuminuria when diagnosed early, and in some cases improve kidney function. This study underscores the critical importance of early detection and aggressive intervention in preventing complications of kidney disease.

Other tests are important too. For example, you should be tested annually for serum creatinine if you have type 1 or type 2 diabetes.

Preventing Nephropathy The key to preventing kidney disease is to maintain tight glucose control and markedly improve your blood pressure. Both the Diabetes Control and Complications Trial (DCCT) in the United States and the United Kingdom Prospective Diabetes Study groups have shown clearly that if you keep your blood sugar close to normal, you can preserve your kidney function and prevent progression to more advanced forms of kidney disease. There are numerous treatment options, depending on the stage of your kidney disease and the results of your annual screening:

- Treat and control high blood pressure. High blood pressure can accelerate the rate at which the disease progresses. Even a mild rise in blood pressure can quickly make kidney disease worsen.
- In the presence of microalbuminuria, your doctor will prescribe drug therapy, either angiotensin converting enzymes (ACE) inhibitors or angiotensin receptor blockers (ARBs) (except during pregnancy). Both drugs are used for controlling high blood pressure and preventing kidney disease in people with diabetes. ACE inhibitors block the production of angiotensin II, a chemical the body produces to raise blood pressure. ARBs block the action of angiotensin II. Both drugs have shown great promise in reducing the risk of kidney disease in diabetics. If for some reason, you cannot tolerate these drugs, your doctor will prescribe a different type of drug therapy. Again, controlling your blood pressure is a very key factor.
- Follow a low-protein diet. Excessive protein seems to increase how hard the kidneys must work. A low-protein diet can improve measures of kidney function.
- Maintain good glucose control. This is key and is particularly important in the early forms of nephropathy.

Treating Nephropathy When kidney disease is caught later, end-stage renal disease, or ESRD, usually follows. ESRD means that the kidneys are failing and can no longer function. Each year in the United States, more than twenty thousand people with diabetes are diagnosed with ESRD. It is treated with kidney dialysis, or through a kidney transplant.

NEUROPATHY

Diabetic neuropathy is a type of nerve damage that happens in people who have diabetes. This damage makes it hard for their nerves to carry messages to the brain and other parts of the body. It can cause numbness (loss of sensation), painful tingling in parts of the body, poor digestion, loss of bladder or bowel control, and impotence. About 60 to 70 percent of people with diabetes have some form of nerve damage.

There are two types of neuropathy:

Distal symmetric polyneuropathy (DPN) is the most common form of diabetic neuropathy and most often develops in the feet, but can also affect the nerves in your arms, hands, and legs. Sensations of pain or tingling are common symptoms, but as the nerve damage progresses, it may lead to poor muscle control and ulcers.

Autonomic neuropathy is a group of symptoms caused by damage to nerves supplying parts of the body that regulate blood pressure, sweating, the eyes, the heart, bowel function, bladder function, and sexual function. Autonomic neuropathy affects internal organs, causing problems with digestion, respiratory function, urination, sexual response, and vision.

Screening for Neuropathy If you have type 1 or type 2 diabetes, be screened annually for DPN. Your doctor will use a variety of simple clinical tests to assess your nerve function. These tests include vibration testing, which uses a special tuning fork to bring out malfunctions of large nerve fibers; temperature testing, using a warm or cold item; or light touch testing or a pinprick test to assess sensation. Screening for automatic neuropathy should begin as soon as you're diagnosed with type 2 diabetes and every five years after you've been diagnosed with type 1 diabetes.

Preventing Neuropathy Diabetic neuropathy occurs in diabetes when your blood sugar level is higher than normal and remains so over time. High blood sugar levels damage the blood vessels and nerves. That's why if you don't control (or can't control) your blood sugar very well, you are at a greater risk of developing diabetic neuropathy. As with all diabetic complications, the most important way to prevent or delay the progression of this complication is to keep your blood sugar under control.

Treating DPN The first step managing DPN is to aim for optimal blood sugar control as assessed with the A1c test. Your doctor can also prescribe certain medications to help alleviate any painful symptoms of DPN, and these are listed in the chart on the following page. It is important to note that many of

Drugs Used to Treat Symptoms of DPN

Class of Drugs	Name (Generic/Brand)	How They Work
Tricyclic drugs	Amitriptyline (Elavil) Nortriptyline (Pamelor, Aventyl) Imipramine (Tofranil)	Increases levels of chemicals in the brain to relieve pain.
Anticonvulsants	Gabapentin (Neurontin) Carbamazepine (Tegretol) Pregabalin (Lyrica)	Calms electrical activity in the brain.
Serotonin and norepinephrine reuptake inhibitor	Duloxetine (Cymbalta)	Helps manage neuropathic pain by restoring the balance of certain naturally occurring chemicals in the brain.
Topical pain reliever	Capsaicin cream	Thought to decrease the amount of a certain substance (substance P) that transmits pain in the body.

these agents, particularly the older agents, *may not be that effective and may have substantial side effects.* It will be important to discuss the side effects of the agents with your physician.

Treating Autonomic Neuropathy Your doctor can use a wide variety of agents to treat the symptoms of autonomic neuropathy, including a drug called metoclopramide (Reglan) if your stomach has become paralyzed due to nerve damage (a condition called gastroparesis) and several medications for bladder and erectile dysfunction. Although they do not change the progression of the disease process, they improve your quality of life by relieving symptoms.

FOOT CARE

Amputation and foot ulcers are the most common consequences of diabetic neuropathy and major causes of disability in people with diabetes. Recognizing foot problems early and managing them can prevent these complications. Your doctor will perform a comprehensive foot examination at least once a year; however, you should examine your own feet every day. Here are some other ways to protect your feet:

- Keep your blood sugar level as close to normal as possible. Follow your program of diet and exercise, and take your diabetes medicine, if your doctor prescribes it.
- Notify your doctor at the first sign of redness, swelling, pain that does not go away, or numbness or tingling in any part of your foot.
- Keep feet clean by washing daily, and be sure to dry your feet well, too, especially between the toes.
- Proper nail and skin care is needed. Patients may need to see a foot care specialist who can assist in cutting nails, debriding calluses, selecting appropriate footwear, and providing the education on proper care of feet.

Macrovascular Complications

HEART DISEASE

If you have diabetes, you run a high risk for having a heart attack or a stroke. In fact, heart disease is one of the leading causes of diabetes-related death. With diabetes, you often have accelerated atherosclerosis, or a buildup of plaque in your arteries, which develops faster than in people without diabetes who have similar risk factors. You may also have an increase in thrombosis, the formation or presence of a clot of coagulated blood in a blood vessel.

A contributing factor to heart disease in people with diabetes is an abnormal profile of blood fats. People with type 2 diabetes, for example, typically have elevated triglycerides. If you have diabetes, strive to keep your triglycerides below 150. You can do this by following a low-fat diet, staying physically active, and maintaining proper weight and glucose control. If you smoke, get help to quit.

Additionally, people with type 2 diabetes frequently have lower-than-optimal levels of high-density cholesterol (HDL), often referred to as the "good cholesterol" because a high level of it protects against heart attack. If your HDL cholesterol is lower than 40, work to raise it. There are many things you can do: exercising, maintaining a healthy weight, quitting smoking, and taking cholesterol-regulating medication if your physician prescribes it.

One of the more important issues related to lipids with diabetes is treating the LDL ("bad" cholesterol). Unfortunately, LDL levels may be normal in individuals with type 2 diabetes, and as such, may go untreated. However, studies have clearly shown that people with type 2 diabetes may need to be placed on a drug, called a statin, to lower the LDL well below currently recommended levels. Specifically, studies have shown that these drugs exert beneficial effects in type 2 diabetics *regardless of the level of the LDL, even if the LDL is considered normal.* So, your doctor may prescribe this medication to you regardless of your level of bad cholesterol. A discussion with your physician on this topic is of utmost importance.

Screening Screening for heart disease involves having a comprehensive medical examination, checking blood pressure, and doing blood work. You should be tested for lipid disorders at least annually and more often if needed to achieve goals.

For most people with diabetes, target levels are:

- LDL cholesterol: Less than 100 mg/dl if you don't have overt heart disease. However, as stated above, studies have shown that reducing LDL levels well below this value may be beneficial, and individuals with type 2 diabetes with "normal" LDL levels appear to benefit from the use of statins. However, if you have had heart disease such as a prior heart attack, the level should be lower and your doctor may suggest a value less than 70 mg/dl.
- HDL cholesterol: Ideally, the higher the good cholesterol the better, but attempt to raise the HDL to greater than 40 mg/dl for men and greater than 50 mg/dl for women.
- Triglycerides: less than 150 mg/dl.

In addition to monitoring blood pressure and blood fats, your doctor may screen for the presence of a molecule called C-reactive protein (CRP). Research suggests that inflammation, the way the body responds to injury, may be important in promoting arteriosclerosis. High levels in the blood of CRP, an inflammatory marker, is associated with heart disease. However, there is no specific treatment for CRP, but treating other conditions such as obesity, elevated glucose, and abnormal lipids will lower the CRP.

Treating Heart Disease If you have heart disease, you'll want to make some modifications in your lifestyle: reduce saturated fat, trans fat (an unhealthy fat found in margarine and processed foods), and cholesterol intake; lose weight

Common Cholesterol-Lowering Medications

Class of Drugs	Name (Generic/Brand)	How They Work
Statins	Atorvastatin calcium (Lipitor) Pravastatin (Pravachol) Simvastatin (Zocor) Rosuvastatin (Crestor) Fluvastatin (Lescol)	Lowers cholesterol by blocking an enzyme in the liver. Your body uses this enzyme to make cholesterol. When less cholesterol is produced, the liver uses up more of it from the blood, thereby lowering levels in your blood. May be indicated in individuals with diabetes regardless of "bad" cholesterol level.
Selective cholesterol-absorption inhibitors	Ezetimibe (Zetia)	Works in the digestive tract to inhibit the absorption of cholesterol. This reduces the amount of intestinal cholesterol delivered to the liver, which reduces the amount of cholesterol in the liver and blood.
Bile acid resins	Cholestyramine (Questran, Questran Light) Colestipol (Colestid) Colesevelam HCl (WelChol)	Binds to bile acids, which are made by breaking down cholesterol, in the intestine. This prevents their absorption, and the cholestyramine/bile acid mixture is eliminated in the stool. To compensate for this loss of bile acids, the liver increases the conversion of cholesterol to bile acids. The conversion reduces the cholesterol in the body, and the levels of cholesterol drop in the blood.
Fibrates	Gemfibrozil (Lopid) Fenofibrate (Tricor)	Reduces blood triglycerides by increasing the activity of enzymes that clear triglycerides from the blood; also reduces the production of cholesterol by the liver.
Prescription vitamin therapy	Nicotinic acid, niacin (Niaspan)	Reduces elevated levels of triglycerides raising low HDL.

if you need to; and increase your physical activity. If you haven't been able to achieve your lipid goals with lifestyle changes alone, your doctor will probably prescribe cholesterol-lowering drugs and/or blood pressure medication, particularly if other cardiovascular risk factors are present. Remember, however, your doctor should strongly consider putting you on a drug called a statin, regardless of your cholesterol levels. The table on page 50 lists common cholesterol-lowering medications and how they work.

Another preventive measure is aspirin therapy (75 to 162 milligrams a day) if you have diabetes with a history of heart trouble. Why aspirin? Aspirin is an antiplatelet drug, meaning that it prevents platelets, tiny clotting substances in the blood, from abnormally clumping together in a process called platelet aggregation. Platelet aggregation triggers the formation of dangerous blood clots that can cause a heart attack by obstructing a blood vessel and shutting off oxygen and nutrients to the heart muscle. Doctors are prescribing aspirin in people with type 1 and type 2 diabetes if they are forty years old or older or if they have additional risk factors for heart disease, including family history, high blood pressure, smoking, abnormal lipids, or more than normal amounts of protein in the urine. Of course, not everyone should take aspirin. Do not take aspirin if you're allergic to aspirin, have a stomach ulcer or active liver disease, or are taking anticlotting drugs (aspirin may increase their action). Don't arbitrarily start taking aspirin either. Do so only under your doctor's orders and guidance.

A comprehensive program of all or most of these measures does wonders in forestalling diabetic-related heart complications. Take the case of Al, for example, who was diagnosed with glucose intolerance and elevated LDL ("bad" cholesterol) that was hovering around 135mg/dl. The sixty-year-old stockbroker was also overweight, with a BMI of 32—probably brought on by his sedentary lifestyle and high-calorie lunches with clients or fast food at his desk. Exercise for him was "something other people did."

One afternoon, Al felt discomfort in his chest, along with sweating and nausea. "I felt like someone was stepping on my chest," he later recalled. He was evaluated in the emergency room and diagnosed as having a heart attack. He was admitted to the hospital, and during a cardiac catherization, a stent was placed in one of his coronary arteries to maintain blood flow. A stent is a device placed inside a blood vessel to provide support and keep the vessel open.

"My doctor told me this has been coming for years and occurred because I had risk factors like abnormal glucose, high cholesterol, obesity, and didn't exercise," Al recalls.

Although Al can't reverse the damage to his heart, he can control these risk factors with diet, exercise, and medication, and hopefully stave off the possibility of a another heart attack. As he puts it, "I went to cardiac rehab, and am now walking actively. I make healthy choices for meals. I have lost twenty pounds. I take my cholesterol medicine faithfully, and my bad cholesterol is now less than 80mg/dl. My glucose is also normal. Also, something as simple as aspirin, which thins my blood, is also considered a lifesaver. I now have a second chance on life."

HYPERTENSION (HIGH BLOOD PRESSURE)

Approximately 60 to 65 percent of people with diabetes have high blood pressure, meaning a reading above 140/90. High blood pressure increases the workload of your heart and arteries. If it continues for a long time, your cardiovascular system may not function properly. Blood vessels of the brain, heart, and kidneys can become damaged, resulting in a stroke, heart failure, or kidney failure. High blood pressure may also increase the risk of heart attack. These problems are less likely to occur if blood pressure is controlled.

Screening In diabetes, high blood pressure is linked to the development of serious complications, including stroke, nephropathy, and retinopathy. Tight blood pressure control is vital to reducing complications and their often life-threatening consequences. If you have diabetes, your blood pressure needs to be 130/80 or lower. You can check this periodically with a home blood pressure monitor, and it should be checked during every routine diabetes visit.

Preventing Hypertension If you have mild to moderate hypertension, make day-to-day changes in your lifestyle. For example:

- Improve your glucose control.
- Do not smoke cigarettes or use tobacco products. Smoking raises your blood pressure and puts you more at risk of heart attack and stroke.
- Work on losing weight, if you are overweight.
- Get more exercise, at least thirty minutes a day several times a week. This can include simple activities like walking the dog, walking in the park, or gardening.
- Modify your dietary intake of salt.

Treating Hypertension If lifestyle changes have not lowered your blood pressure, your physician will probably add some sort of drug treatment to your routine. ACE inhibitors, angiotensin receptor blockers (ARBs), beta-blockers, calcium channel blockers, and diuretics are commonly prescribed drugs that lower blood pressure. Sometimes, you may have to take two or more drugs to reduce your blood pressure. Your doctor will select the best form of drug therapy based on your health and the results of your physical examinations. Commonly prescribed blood pressure medications are described below.

Common Anti-Hypertension Medications

Class of Drugs	Name (Generic/Brand)	How They Work
Angiotensin converting enzyme (ACE) inhibitors	Quinapril hydrochloride (Accupril) Captopril (Capoten) Benazepril (Lotensin) Fosinopril (Monopril) Lisinopril (Prinivil, Zestril) Enalapril (Vasotec)	Block the production of angiotensin II, a chemical the body produces to raise blood pressure. Very effective to reduce albuminuria in individuals with diabetes.
Angiotensin II receptor blockers	Losartan (Cozaar) Valsartan (Diovan) Irbesartan (Avapro) Candesartan cilexetil (Atacand)	Block the action of certain chemicals that narrow the blood vessels, allowing blood to flow more easily through your body, which lowers blood pressure. Effective to reduce albuminuria.
Beta-blockers	Propranolol (Inderal) Atenolol (Tenormin) Metoprolol tartrate (Lopressor) Acebutolol hydrochloride (Sectral) Betaxolol hydrochloride (Kerlone) Bisoprolol (Zebeta) Hydrochlorothiazide and bisoprolol (Ziac) Carteolol (Cartrol) Carvedilol (Coreg) Labetalol hydrochloride (Normodyne) Labetalol Injection (Trandate)	Decrease the force and rate of heart contractions.

(continued)

Common Anti-Hypertension Medications
(continued)

Class of Drugs	Name (Generic/Brand)	How They Work
Beta-blockers *(continued)*	Nadolol (Corgard) Penbutolol (Levatol) Pindolol (Visken) Timolol (Blocadren)	
Thiazide diuretics	Bendroflumethiazide (Naturetin) Benzthiazide (Aquatag, Exna, Marazide) Chlorothiazide (Diuril) Cyclothiazide (Anhydron) Hydrochlorothiazide (Esidrix, HydroDiuril) Hydroflumethiazide (Diucardin, Saluron) Methyclothiazide (Aquatensen, Enduron) Polythiazide (Renese) Trichlormethiazide (Metahydrin, Naqua)	Contain a form of thiazide, a diuretic that prompts your body to produce and eliminate more urine. May be used with other blood pressure agents to enhance the effect on blood pressure lowering.
Alpha-blockers	Doxazosin mesylate (Cardura) Prazosin (Minipress) Terazosin (Hytrin) Doxazosin mesilate (Apa-Doxazosin, Doxaloc, Gen-Doxazosin, Med-Doxazosin)	Block the effect of adrenaline, a hormone released by the body in response to stress. Too much over-excites the circulatory system, causing an increase in blood pressure. Alpha-blockers cause the muscles in the artery walls to relax.
Calcium channel blockers	Nifedipine (Adalat) Verapamil (Calan, Isoptin, Verelan) Diltiazem (Cardizen) Amlodipine (Norvasc) Nifedipine (Procardia, Procardia XL) Bepridil hydrochloride (Vascor) Diltiazem hydrochloride (Tiazac) Felodipine (Plendil) Isradipine (DynaCirc) Nicardipine (Cardene) Nimodipine (Nimotop) Nisoldipine (Sular)	Relax the arteries and reduce resistance to blood flow.

STROKE

Common in diabetic patients, stroke is a disturbance to the brain's blood supply, caused by a blood clot or by a ruptured blood vessel that bleeds into the brain. One of the most important measures to take is controlling your blood pressure. The UKPDS study showed that when blood pressure is driven down, the result is a 44 percent reduction in the risk of fatal and nonfatal strokes. Additionally, to prevent stroke, you must stop smoking if you're a smoker, follow a low-fat diet, control your body weight, and stay active. Your doctor may also prescribe blood pressure medication to reduce your risk of stroke.

PREVENTING COMPLICATIONS: A MEDICAL CHECKLIST

Use this simple checklist, and keep it handy, for actions to take to reduce your risk of complications from diabetes.

- Know your hemoglobin A1c level. Keep your level below 7 percent. The lower the better.
- Monitor your glucose daily.
- Have a lipid panel (total cholesterol, HDL, LDL, and triglycerides) to check heart disease risk: once a year.
- Monitor your blood pressure at home and during routine diabetic visits.
- Foot check for sores or ulcers (performed by your physician): at least once a year.
- Eye screening for retinopathy, a condition that can lead to blindness: once a year.
- Have your urine tested for protein: once a year.

*

Preventing diabetic complications demands more of a commitment than many other illnesses. But if you work on your lifestyle, blood sugar, blood pressure, and cholesterol, and other aspects of your health, your chances of staying healthy can only improve. Staying aware of any changes in your body, and reporting them to your physician, is vital too. Do the best you can, and there is nothing that can stop you from leading a full, active, and healthy life.

Yes, particularly if you have diabetic nerve damage, or are taking certain medications that are known to affect sexual response, such as blood pressure medicine, certain lipid-lowering drugs, and antidepressants. For example, men can have trouble maintaining an erection and ejaculating. Women can have trouble with sexual response and vaginal lubrication. Several options are now available for treating these problems: sexual therapy, oral agents for men, vaginal lubricants, and other therapies (talk to your doctor, gynecologist, or urologist).

＊

ASK DR. CEFALU: CAN SOMEONE WITH DIABETES DIE
IF THE DISEASE ISN'T TREATED?

The short answer is—yes. Truthfully, and I don't mean to alarm anyone, uncontrolled diabetes can lead to very serious and often life-threatening complications, which include blindness, kidney disease, lower-limb amputations, heart disease, and stroke. Practically every body system can become damaged. Thus, someone's life span, if diabetes is not controlled, can be cut short by a number of complications. But this does not have to happen. You can control diabetes by changing your lifestyle through nutrition, exercise, self-monitoring of glucose levels, medical supervision, and medication.

＊

ASK DR. CEFALU: HOW DOES MAINTAINING A HEALTHY BLOOD
PRESSURE LEVEL HELP PEOPLE WITH DIABETES STAY HEALTHY?

High blood pressure, or hypertension, is very common in diabetes; approximately 70 percent of adults with diabetes have high blood pressure or must use prescription medications to manage it. Maintaining normal blood pressure— less than 130/80—helps prevent damage to the eyes, kidneys, heart, and blood vessels. In general, for every 10 mm reduction in systolic blood pressure (the first number in the reading), the risk for any complication related to diabetes goes down by approximately 12 percent. Proper nutrition, medications, and regular exercise can help you normalize your blood pressure.

＊

If you smoke and have diabetes, you have additional—and serious—risks to your health. Smoking damages your blood vessels. If you quit smoking, you'll lower your risk for heart attack, stroke, nerve disease, kidney disease, and oral disease.

＊

Yes. When your cholesterol is too high, the linings of large blood vessels will become damaged. This sets the stage for heart disease and stroke, two of the biggest health problems for people with diabetes. If you maintain healthy cholesterol and triglyceride levels, you help prevent these diseases, as well as circulation problems, also an issue if you have diabetes. Have your cholesterol checked at least once a year. Total cholesterol should be under 200; LDL ("bad" cholesterol) should be under 100; HDL ("good" cholesterol) should be above 40 in men and above 50 in women; and triglycerides should be under 150. If you have diabetes or prior heart disease, your doctor may want to treat your LDL even to lower levels. Healthy eating, medications, and physical activity can help you reach your cholesterol targets. If you keep your cholesterol levels under control, you can reduce the risk of cardiovascular complications by 20 to 50 percent.

＊

Part 2

A Lifestyle Prescription for Preventing and Managing Diabetes

4

Making the Most of Your Food

IF YOU'VE BEEN CONFUSED OVER WHAT
to eat and not eat, I have two very simple pieces of advice: number one, go
for pure foods, not processed foods; and number two, gravitate toward low-
fat foods.

A number of studies, including the ones I'll tell you about here, have con-
vincingly shown that most people with diabetes can significantly lower their
blood sugar levels, often within weeks, by following a nutritious diet that's low
in fat and calories and high in the fiber contained in nonprocessed foods like
fruits, vegetables, and whole grains. This approach is also good for those of
you who need to lose weight.

Why are these two strategies such a big deal?

Eating natural, unprocessed fiber-rich foods plays a key role by helping stabilize your blood sugar levels. When foods are eaten without their normal complement of fiber—I'm talking about refined, processed, or packaged foods—
blood sugar levels can quickly rise. Normally a surge of insulin counteracts

this, but if you have diabetes, your body doesn't make enough insulin, or it doesn't respond to insulin properly. If you consume refined foods, drinks, snacks, and foods high in calories and simple sugars but low in fiber, you may experience too many ups in blood sugar levels. Thus, you'll want to choose mostly whole foods, relying on fewer highly processed ones. Grains, fruits, vegetables, and legumes contain fiber, vitamins, and minerals, and along with lean proteins, should be the mainstay of any diet. Processed foods should be limited, and the focus placed on natural and fresh choices. Processed foods tend to be high in fat; often high in sodium, which can be detrimental to blood pressure; and sometimes high in calories, which of course leads to weight gain.

I'm going to give you two different diets—both based on these principles and both taken from the very latest nutritional research into diabetes. These diets have been proven, hands down, to help you achieve tighter control of blood sugar levels, especially when coupled with other lifestyle changes and sometimes medication, and therefore represent an ideal way to prevent or manage diabetes. Once you get used to eating the "real food" on these diets, discovering how much better it tastes and makes you feel, you'll never be able to go back to your old eating habits again. Using either of these diets, you will also:

- Protect your heart by improving your lipid (cholesterol and triglycerides) profile and controlling your blood pressure.
- Help achieve and maintain a reasonable weight. A reasonable weight is one that is achievable and sustainable over time and includes a dietary pattern that provides proper nutrients, including fiber. You'll find that eating unprocessed food will help you control your weight easily because of that fiber. Fiber makes you feel full, so you don't overeat. And fiber helps move food through your system more efficiently. As a result, you'll be able to control your weight more easily. If you are overweight with type 2 diabetes and *not* taking medication, you'll want to control both your weight and glucose. The diets in this chapter help you do that.
- Manage or prevent complications of diabetes—because the low-fat, un-processed food approach is an effective way to stabilize blood sugar, and help tighten its control. As a result, you'll enhance your overall health and have a better quality of life.

Just by reducing consumption of processed food, you can help to accomplish all this and become considerably healthier. A good example is Candace, a thirty-nine-year-old bank manager. She was diagnosed with type 2 diabetes, high blood pressure, high cholesterol, and obesity (she weighed 175 pounds at five feet three). Her father had died from complications related to diabetes; Candace did not want to endure the same fate. She was scared.

Candace's fortuitous decision to make lifestyle changes quickly may have helped her dodge the often-deadly complications of diabetes. With the help of a registered dietitian who helped her get past obstacles to healthier habits, Candace started following the research-backed dietary guidelines you'll learn about here. She reduced her fat intake to less than 30 percent of her total calories, she boosted her intake of fruits, vegetables, and whole grains, and she made it a point to eat more fiber. She banished snack foods, sweets, soft drinks, and all processed foods from her home. Candace was religious about her new diet and kept a diary of what she ate, her portion sizes, and the fat content of her meals. She fit exercise into her lifestyle too, with some easy-does-it activity—walking thirty minutes most days of the week.

Over time, she has lost—and kept off—twenty pounds. Her blood pressure and cholesterol have normalized, and her blood sugar readings indicate excellent glucose control. In effect, Candace has addressed her diabetes and essentially stopped it.

When you eat low-fat, natural, unrefined foods like Candace did, there's no need to feel singled out either. The way you should eat is exactly the way everyone in this country should eat for good health. Your family can benefit from following these diets too. So if you're willing to tweak your nutrition a bit, the rewards are well worth the effort. The earlier you start making good nutrition a habit, the greater your ability to stop this disease.

Nutrition and Diabetes

The two diets with the most science behind them are those used in the Diabetes Prevention Program (DPP) and the Dietary Approaches to Stop Hypertension (DASH) trials. Both are built around the two key strategies I've already introduced: natural, unprocessed foods, and low-fat foods. What these diets have in common is that they are built around healthy choices and nutrients that help prevent or manage diabetes.

The DPP diet focused primarily on preventing diabetes, while the DASH diet was specifically designed to reduce high blood pressure, but was also found to help control diabetes, improve blood fats, and reduce cancer risk. Before we look at the diets, let's review the bigger nutritional picture.

Carbohydrates

Carbohydrates are present in vegetables, fruits, grains, cereals, breads, sugars, and to some extent, dairy foods. There are two general classifications of carbohydrates: simple and complex. Simple carbohydrates, found in sweets, white bread, cakes, candy, and other processed foods with added sugars, are quickly digested by your body and stimulate a rapid spike in blood glucose. Complex carbohydrates, on the other hand, particularly those rich in fiber, do not normally elicit the same kind of quick response. The speed at which glucose is released into the bloodstream by a particular carbohydrate is termed its glycemic index. I'll discuss this later in the chapter.

You'll want to choose natural, unprocessed carbohydrates, typically the complex ones, because they are high in many nutrients. One of these is fiber, the material that gives strength and support to plant tissues, as well as texture. Although it is primarily made up of carbohydrates, fiber does not have a lot of usable calories. The beauty of fiber, though, is that foods containing it break down into glucose more gradually. This means that glucose is absorbed more slowly into your bloodstream. Also, fiber keeps your stomach from emptying too quickly and helps you feel full.

There are two types of fiber in natural, unprocessed foods: soluble and insoluble. Insoluble fiber adds bulk to your diet, helps maintain intestinal health, and may help in preventing some cancers. It does not dissolve in water and is mainly found in vegetables (particularly the skin), fruit pulp, and the bran layer of grains. Soluble fiber attracts water during digestion and is found in oat bran, seeds, beans, and certain fruits and vegetables. The current recommendation for fiber is 20 to 35 grams daily. The chart on the following pages lists a number of fiber-rich foods worth adding to your diet.

Protein

Protein from any number of sources—plant protein or animal protein—is part of a healthy diet to prevent or manage diabetes. Generally, its role is to support the growth, repair, and maintenance of body tissues. The amount of

Fiber Content of Common Foods

Legumes	Typical serving size	Total fiber (grams)
Lentils, cooked	½ cup	7.8
Black beans, cooked	½ cup	7.5
Lima beans, baby, cooked	½ cup	7.0
Baked beans, canned, no meat	½ cup	5.2

Vegetables	Typical serving size	Total fiber (grams)
Peas, green, cooked	½ cup	4.4
Artichoke, cooked	1 medium	6.5
Brussels sprouts, frozen, cooked	1 cup	6.4
Turnip greens, boiled	1 cup	5.0
Potato, baked with skin	1 medium	3.8
Corn, yellow, cooked	½ cup	2.3
Popcorn, air-popped	3 cups	3.5
Tomato, red, raw	1 large whole	2.2
Carrot, raw	1 medium	1.7

Grains, cereal & pasta	Typical serving size	Total fiber (grams)
Spaghetti, plain	1 cup	2.5
Spaghetti, whole wheat	1 cup	6.3
Bran flakes	¾ cup	5.3
Oatmeal	½ cup	2.0
Bread, white	1-oz. slice	0.7
Bread, rye	1-oz. slice	1.6
Bread, whole wheat	1-oz. slice	1.9
Bread, mixed-grain	1-oz. slice	1.8
Bread, cracked-wheat	1-oz. slice	1.6
Rice, white	½ cup	0.3
Rice, brown	½ cup	1.8

Fruits	Typical serving size	Total fiber (grams)
Pear, raw	1 medium	5.5
Figs, dried	2 medium	1.6

(continued)

Fiber Content of Common Foods
(continued)

Fruits	Typical serving size	Total fiber (grams)
Blueberries, raw	1 cup	3.6
Apple, raw with skin	1 medium	3.3
Banana, raw	1 medium	3.1
Strawberries, whole	1 cup	2.9
Peaches, raw	1 medium	2.2
Orange	1 medium	3.1
Apricots, dried	5 halves	1.3
Raisins	1.5-oz. box	1.6

protein you need daily depends on your diabetic condition. Your doctor may recommend a protein intake of as much as 20 percent of your daily calories. However, if your doctor detects signs of nephropathy (kidney disease), then your protein intake may be lowered.

Some studies suggest that the protein coming from animal sources is more of a problem in kidney disease than that from vegetable sources. But regardless of the source, in diabetic nutrition, protein is an important part of the diet and, when combined with carbohydrates and fat in a meal, helps to maintain a normal blood sugar level.

You'll want to choose lean proteins, those that are low in fat. These include white-meat poultry, fish, and certain cuts of red meat (top round, top loin, round tip, tenderloin, sirloin, or eye of the round). Also, choose low-fat dairy products like skim milk and nonfat yogurt. These foods are also a rich source of calcium.

Fat

In diabetic nutrition, a lot of attention is paid to carbohydrates, which are certainly important. But based on recent research, more emphasis should be on controlling fat in your diet. It may sound like old news, but low-fat diets are vital for managing your health if you have prediabetes or diabetes.

By low-fat diets, I do not mean a diet that drastically slashes all fats. We

Good Fats

Dietary Fats	Sources	Function	Role in Diabetes
Polyunsaturated fats	Corn, soybean, sesame, some fish	Provide energy; help to lower bad cholesterol and may increase good cholesterol levels.	May be protective against heart and vascular system complications.
Monounsaturated fats	Olive, canola, peanut oils; avocado, some fish	Provide energy; tend to lower bad cholesterol and may increase good cholesterol levels; may reduce triglycerides.	Improve lipid profiles as well as glycemic control (helping to improve your diabetic condition).
Omega-3 fats	Flaxseed oil, canola oil, pumpkin seeds, walnuts, oily fish, including salmon, tuna, sardines, rainbow trout	Polyunsaturated fats that reduce abnormal heart rhythms, improve blood clotting regulation; lower triglycerides.	May reduce heart disease risk. May reduce blood pressure by small but significant amounts.
Omega-6 fats	Many vegetable oils, seeds, nuts; borage oil, black currant seed oil.	Polyunsaturated fats that are involved in cellular health.	May assist nerve function.

now know that there are good and bad types of fat. The good fats—found in foods like fish, olive oil, avocados, and many nuts—actually improve cholesterol levels in your blood and may significantly reduce the risk of heart disease. Bad fats are detrimental, and there are two types. Saturated fats—typically found in red meat, butter, ice cream, and tropical oils—increase your risk of heart disease by elevating total cholesterol levels in the body. Trans fats—found primarily in processed foods, such as stick margarines and many commercially baked or fried foods—may elevate LDL ("bad" cholesterol) and lower beneficial HDL ("good" cholesterol). By reducing consumption of processed foods, you'll automatically decrease intake of trans fats. Food labels now contain information on trans fats.

According to current recommendations, 25 to 35 percent of your daily calories should come from fat, and less than 10 percent of those calories should be from saturated fats.

It is also important to watch your intake of another type of fat, cholesterol, from food. Try to keep your intake of cholesterol under 300 milligrams daily. This is fairly easy to do if you cut back on cholesterol-containing foods like red meats and limit your egg consumption to around three eggs a week.

Getting Started

That's the end of my nutrition overview. Now I'd like to introduce you to the two diets that can help you stop prediabetes and control diabetes. You have the flexibility of choosing either one, or switching back and forth between the two. The key is to try to stick to your diet as closely as possible, and later in this chapter I'll give you some tools and tips for doing so. I think you'll find both diets easy to follow, because you won't feel hungry or deprived. And in the chapter that follows, you'll find some delicious recipes that will help you stay the course.

A Nutrition Prescription for Stopping Prediabetes

The first diet is effective for treating prediabetes—having higher-than-normal blood sugar levels. This is something you cannot ignore, since it puts you at higher risk for developing type 2 diabetes and heart disease. This diet comes from an important study on how to prevent progression to diabetes: the DPP. This major clinical research study focused on whether either improvements in diet and exercise (lifestyle), compared to taking the oral diabetes drug metformin (Glucophage), could prevent or delay the onset of type 2 diabetes in people with prediabetes. Participants ate less fat and fewer calories, exercised for one hundred fifty minutes a week, and set goals of losing 7 percent of their body weight and maintaining that weight loss. The results of the study found that these measures, particularly modest weight loss and regular exercise, can prevent or delay type 2 diabetes.

Specifically, people participating in the DPP plan, called the Lifestyle Balance Program, did the following:

- Used the government's familiar Food Guide Pyramid to make wise food choices.
- Cut their intake of dietary fat by reducing their intake of high-fat foods, eating smaller portions of high-fat foods, and choosing lower-fat foods.
- Reduced their daily calories to lose weight.
- Weighed themselves regularly.
- Changed their eating behavior by following a regular pattern of meals, eating more slowly, and serving smaller portions of food.
- Learned how to manage their hunger by removing high-calorie, processed foods from their environment.
- Learned how to eat out in restaurants and make healthy choices.

Although participants in the DPP met with a lifestyle counselor, usually a dietitian, and completed sixteen lessons devoted to lifestyle, it is likely that with motivation you can do it on your own. To access the participants' actual educational materials, visit http://www.bsc.gwu.edu/dpp/lifestyle/dpp_acor.html.

Even though you weren't a part of the DPP study, you can easily apply it to your own life in order to manage prediabetes or diabetes. The section below shows you how to take the lessons learned in the DPP and use them to plan your daily menus.

Follow the Food Guide Pyramid

As I noted, the DPP used the Food Guide Pyramid, a meal-planning system developed in 1994 by the United States Department of Agriculture (USDA). It has since been refined and updated. The newest version is called MyPyramid, and it is available online at www.mypyramid.gov. It offers you a personal eating plan with the foods and amounts that are right for you and places healthy food choices in various food groups. As the DPP participants did, you can use the pyramid's recommendations to plan your meals based on the following guidelines:

Reduce Your Fat Intake

Fat is essentially the most fattening thing we eat and contains more than twice the calories as the same amount of sugar, starch, or protein. Fortunately,

Food Group and Number of Daily Servings	Choose these foods:	Avoid and cut back on these foods (high-fat and high-sugar foods):
Breads, cereals, rice, pastas (6 to 11 servings)	• 1 slice whole wheat bread or tortilla • ½ whole wheat bagel, whole wheat English muffin, whole wheat pita bread • ½ cup cooked whole-grain cereal, whole wheat pasta, bulgur, rice (preferably brown) • ¾ cup dry cereal (preferably a fiber-rich cereal)	• Granola-type cereals (except low-fat type) • Croissants, sweet rolls, doughnuts, muffins, Danish pastry, biscuits, high-fat crackers, regular tortilla chips, fried tortillas
Vegetables (3 to 5 servings)	• 1 cup raw vegetables • ½ cup cooked vegetables or vegetable juice	• Fried vegetables • Vegetables with butter/margarine, cream, or cheese sauces • Olives, avocados (good kind of fat if you need some extra fat)
Fruits (2 to 4 servings)	• 1 small fresh fruit • 1 cup chopped fresh fruit	• High in sugar: dried fruit, juices or drinks sweetened with sugar, fruit canned in syrup, large amounts of fruit juice • Fruits in pastry (as in pies), coconut
Milk, yogurt, cheese (2 to 3 servings)	• 1 cup skim or 1% milk • 1 cup low- or nonfat yogurt • 2–3 ounces low- or nonfat cheese (<2 grams fat/ounce)	• 2% or whole milk • Regular cheese (>2 grams fat/ounce) • High in sugar: yogurt with added sugar
Meat, poultry, fish, dry beans, eggs (2 to 3 servings)	• 2–3 ounces cooked lean meat, poultry (without skin), or fish • ½ cup tuna, canned in water • ½ cup cooked dry beans, lentils, split peas • 1 egg or ¼ cup egg substitute	• Bacon, sausage, hot dogs, hamburgers, luncheon meats, most red meats (except lean, trimmed cuts) • Chicken or turkey with skin • Tuna canned in oil • Beans cooked in lard or salt pork

(continued)

Food Group and Number of Daily Servings	Choose these foods:	Avoid and cut back on these foods (high-fat and high-sugar foods):
Fats, sweets, alcohol (limit)	Low-fat substitutes: • Low-fat or fat-free margarine, mayonnaise, salad dressings, cream cheese, or sour cream Foods lower in sugar: • All-fruit jams • Diet soft drinks • Lite syrup	• Regular margarine, shortening, lard, oil, butter, mayonnaise, salad dressing, cream cheese, sour cream • Half-and-half, whipped cream • Cakes, cookies, ice cream, candy, cupcakes • Honey, jelly, syrup, sugar • Soft drinks

there are many ways you can cut the bad fat in your diet, and do it easily and automatically. Here are some suggestions recommended by the DPP:

- Figure out how much fat you consume now by writing down everything you eat and drink each day. Include the time you ate them and exactly what you ate. Analyze this record by reading labels or using a fat counter to discover which foods you eat are high in fat, since much of the fat we eat, actually more than half of it, is hidden in foods. Add up the fat you eat during the day.
- Decide on a "fat budget" based on your calorie intake. As an example, if you need to eat only 1,200 calories per day and your desirable percent of calories from fat is 30 percent, then that is [1200 x .3], or 360 calories. One gram of fat has 9 calories, therefore $360 \div 9 = 40$ grams of fat. That would be your goal; just try to get as close to it as you can.
- Replace high-fat foods with lower-fat foods. Select fresh fruit and vegetables for snacks, for example. Serve vegetarian dinners several times a week. Eat fruit for dessert. Try lower-fat substitutes, too, such as low-fat or fat-free margarine and mayonnaise, cheese, salad dressings, or skim or 1% fat milk.

Other tips are listed in the charts that follow.

TIPS FOR REDUCING FAT AND CHOLESTEROL

- Use cooking techniques that require no added fat, such as broiling, grilling, poaching, steaming, or baking.
- Avoid frying foods. Poach, boil, or scramble eggs (or egg whites) with vegetable cooking spray. Microwave, steam, or boil vegetables in a small amount of water, or try stir-frying them.
- Utilize a rack when broiling or baking meat so the juices and fat will drain off. Skim the fat from meat juice before using it to make gravies, sauces, and stews.
- Keep your kitchen well stocked with condiments and various spices to flavor your foods: herbs, spice blends, hot sauce, mustard, and fat-free salsas (if you are trying to lower your sodium, check that salsa label).
- Pour healthy fats such as olive oil or canola oil into a pump spray bottle for cooking on a nonstick skillet or spritzing vegetables. Three pumps equals approximately one teaspoon of oil. Or use vegetable cooking sprays instead of frying with oil.
- At restaurants, have salad dressing served on the side and just dip the fork in the dressing before spearing some salad.
- Use some of the new spray-bottle salad dressings to get all the flavor of high-fat salad dressings but very little of the fat calories.
- Remove most of the fat from a can of soup by putting it in the freezer for ten minutes, removing it, then scooping the fat off the top.
- Microwave vegetables in a small amount of water or fat-free broth.
- Use a diet-friendly marinade such as fat-free salad dressing to tenderize meats.
- To get the leanest and freshest ground beef, have your butcher trim off any visible fat from a round of sirloin steak, then grind the meat fresh.
- Buy lean cuts, such as round, loin, sirloin, or leg.
- For ground beef, put it in a colander after cooking and rinse with hot water.
- Flavor meats with low-fat flavorings, such as barbecue sauce, Tabasco, ketchup, lemon juice, or Worcestershire sauce.
- Remove the skin from chicken; this reduces the fat calories by up to 50 percent. You can, however, leave the skin on during cooking (the fat from the skin won't leach into the meat) and remove it before serving.
- Forgo the butter or margarine on your dinner roll. Instead, try dipping the roll in a tablespoon of extra-virgin olive oil. Unlike butter, olive oil contains very little saturated fat and is loaded with healthy mono-unsaturated fats.
- Avoid any foods with breading; these usually are fried and high in fat.

- Choose low-fat dairy products.
- Eat more fiber, especially the cholesterol-lowering soluble kind found in sources like oats, oat bran, beans, peas, citrus fruits, strawberries, and apples.
- Avoid foods that contain hydrogenated oil, which boosts LDL ("bad" cholesterol) and decreases HDL ("good" cholesterol). Prime culprits are frozen dinners, margarine, cookies, and virtually all commercial snack foods. You are actually checking for saturated and trans fats, so the label is helpful here too. Choose products low in saturated and trans fats.
- Try tofu, roasted soy beans, or soy milk. Soy is a proven cholesterol fighter.
- Select heart-healthy oils. Monounsaturated oils (olive, canola, peanut) are best because they lower LDL but not HDL levels. Polyunsaturated oils (safflower, corn, sunflower, soybean, sesame) reduce both LDL and HDL.
- Try a nutraceutical spread like Benecol or Take Control on your toast. Take Control is now marketed as Promise Activ. If you're on cholesterol-lowering medication, however, check with your health-care provider first.

Using Low-fat Flavorings

To flavor these foods:	Use these low-fat flavorings:
Potatoes, vegetables	Low-fat margarine (small amount), nonfat sour cream, defatted broth, low-fat or fat-free plain yogurt, salsa. Herbs, mustard, lemon juice.
Bread	Nonfat cream cheese, low-fat margarine (small amount), all-fruit jams.
Pancakes	Fruit, low-calorie syrup, unsweetened applesauce, crushed berries.
Salads	Nonfat or low-fat salad dressing, lemon juice, vinegar.
Pasta, rice	Spaghetti sauce without meat or added fat, chopped vegetables, white sauce made with skim or 1% milk and no fat.

Reduce Your Daily Calories to Lose Weight

Calories in food come from fat, starches and sugars, protein, or alcohol, with fat having the highest calories per gram. Calories also measure the energy you use up in daily life activities. Your weight is a result of the balance between food (calories in) and activity (calories out). So at its heart, the rule for losing weight is simple: eat fewer calories than you burn. Here's why: one pound of fat equals about 3,500 calories, so you can lose a pound a week by reducing your daily caloric intake, increasing your physical activity level, or both, by about 500 calories a day. Most women can lose weight on 1,200 calories daily; most men, 1,600 calories. Here is a look at how many calories to cut, either from your diet, through exercise, or both, each day to lose weight:

To lose:	Reduce this amount of calories:
1 pound/week	3,500 calories per week (or 500 calories each day for 7 days)
1½ pounds/week	5,250 calories per week (or 750 calories each day for 7 days)
2 pounds/week	7,000 calories per week (or 1,000 calories each day for 7 days)

Weigh Yourself Regularly

People who are successful at weight management weigh themselves regularly, according to the National Weight Control Registry, a study of more than five thousand who have lost weight and kept it off for a significant period of time. Decide on a regular weighing schedule, and weigh yourself on the same scale and at the same time of the day. Chart your weight beginning with your starting weight, or keep track of your weight loss progress in a notebook.

Monitor Your New Eating Habits

A good idea is to periodically rate your plate. Using the chart on the following page, check one box for every serving you ate on a particular day. The shaded boxes show you the minimum number of servings recommended (from the older version of the Food Guide Pyramid). Monitor yourself like this every few days to see how you're doing.

Modify Your Eating Behavior

Some very simple techniques can help you stick to your eating plan. A regular pattern of meals is important, for example, because it keeps you from getting too hungry and losing control. Try to eat your meals and snacks at the same time each day. Eating slowly is also key, so you can digest your food bet-

Serving Sizes

Bread, cereal, rice, pasta

1 slice whole wheat bread or tortilla; or ½ whole wheat bagel, whole wheat English muffin, or whole wheat pita bread; ½ cup cooked whole-grain cereal, whole wheat pasta, bulgur, rice; ¾ cup dry cereal (preferably fiber-rich cereals such as Fiber One or All-Bran)

Vegetables

1 cup raw vegetables; ½ cup cooked vegetables or vegetable juice

Fruit

1 small fresh fruit; 1 cup chopped fresh fruit

Milk, yogurt, cheese

1 cup skim or 1% milk; 1 cup low- or nonfat yogurt; 2–3 ounces low- or nonfat cheese (<2 grams fat per ounce)

Meat, poultry, fish, dry beans, eggs

2–3 ounces cooked lean meat, poultry, (without skin), or fish; ½ cup tuna, canned in water; ½ cup cooked dry beans, lentils, split peas; 1 egg or ¼ cup egg substitute

Fats, sweets, alcohol (sparingly)

ter, stay aware of what you're eating, and register when you are full. Try pausing between bites of food by putting down your fork and enjoying the taste of your food. Serve yourself smaller portions of food, too. And don't worry about having to clean your plate.

Manage Your Hunger

Try to keep high-fat/high-calorie foods out of your house and workplace. Or at least keep them hidden, since "out of sight is out of mind." Instead, keep lower-fat/calorie choices easy to reach, in sight, and ready to eat. Recommended foods are fresh fruits, raw vegetables (already washed and prepared), diet drinks, sugar-free Jell-O, and sugar-free Popsicles. Limit your eating to one place. When you eat, limit other activities.

Grocery shopping can be the downfall of healthy eating, unless you plan ahead. Here are some shopping tips:

- Make a shopping list ahead of time. Stick to your list.
- Don't go shopping when you're hungry.
- Avoid sections in the store that are tempting to you, if possible.
- Ask the grocery store manager to order low-fat and low-calorie foods you want, if they are not routinely stocked.
- Only use food coupons for low-fat and low-calorie foods, not for high-fat foods.

Make Healthy Choices at Restaurants

Dining out can be a significant challenge for diabetics, people trying to lose weight, and anyone adhering to a specific dietary regimen. In the tables that follow are some tips that were used in the DPP that can help you.

A Nutrition Prescription for Managing Diabetes

One of the healthiest diets today for managing diabetes resulted from a government-funded study called the Dietary Approaches to Stop Hypertension, or DASH. This study looked at the effects of certain dietary patterns on reducing blood pressure. What happened was that the diet was not only effective for controlling blood pressure, it was also found to be an appropriate diet for cardiovascular disease, cancer prevention, and is promoted as one way to help in managing diabetes. This diet is high in protective antioxidants, vitamins, and the electrolytes potassium, calcium, and magnesium.

Specifically, the DASH diet:

- Reduces saturated fat (but includes calcium-rich dairy products that are nonfat or low-fat).
- Recommends monounsaturated oils, such as olive or canola.
- Emphasizes whole grains over processed white flour or pasta products.
- Suggests fresh fruits and vegetables every day. Here is an amazing benefit of switching to unprocessed foods: in one part of the DASH study, people who increased their intake of fruits and vegetables experienced a drop in blood pressure as quickly as two weeks after starting the plan. Many of these foods are rich in potassium and fiber, both of which may help lower blood pressure.
- Advises including nuts, seeds, or legumes (dried beans or peas) daily.
- Stresses choosing modest amounts of lean protein (preferably fish, white-meat poultry, or soy products).
- Recommends no more than 2,300 milligrams of sodium each day.

You can find out more about the entire DASH project by going to the following Web site. It has menus and more information as to how to follow the DASH diet as well: http://www.nhlbi.nih.gov/health/public/heart/hbp/dash/new_dash.pdf.

Here is a guide to planning a diabetes management diet based on the nutritional principles used in the DASH diet:

Eat 6 to 8 Daily Servings of Grains

Most of your choices should come from whole grains because they are the highest in fiber and nutrients. Examples of grains include: whole wheat bread and rolls; whole wheat pasta; whole wheat English muffins; pita bread; bagels; whole-grain cereals; grits; oatmeal; brown rice; air-popped popcorn.

Typical serving sizes include: 1 slice of bread; 1 ounce of dry cereal, or between ½ cup and 1¼ cups, depending on the serving size on the product's Nutrition Facts Label; or ½ cup of cooked rice, pasta, or cereal.

Eat 4 to 5 Daily Servings of Vegetables

Vegetables should be the centerpiece of your diet because they are important sources of protective antioxidants, phytochemicals, minerals, and fiber. Healthy vegetable choices include broccoli, carrots, collards, green beans,

PLAN AHEAD

- Pick carefully where you eat out; call beforehand to ask about low-fat, low-calorie choices.
- Eat less fat and fewer calories during other meals that day to compensate for eating out.
- Eat a little something before you go out, or drink a large, low-calorie beverage in order to help control your hunger. Plan what to order without looking at the menu if that's a possibility.
- Don't drink alcohol before eating. Alcohol stimulates your appetite and lowers your inhibitions, increasing the chance that you'll overindulge.
- For parties or dinner parties, bring something from home that fits your lifestyle to share with others.

TAKE CONTROL

- Ask for what you want, namely low-fat or low-calorie dishes, in the amounts you want.
- Be firm and friendly.
- Ask if foods can be cooked in a different way.
- Don't be afraid to ask for foods that aren't on the menu.
- Order salad dressing, gravy, sauces, or spreads "on the side."
- Ask for less cheese or no cheese.
- Split a main dish or dessert with someone.
- Order a small size (appetizer, senior citizen's, children's size).
- Before or after the meal, have the amount you don't want to eat put in a container to take home.
- Ask that your plate be removed as soon as you finish.

AVOID HIGH-FAT FOOD PREPARATION

Watch out for these high-fat words on menus:
- Au gratin, breaded, buttered or buttery, cheese sauce
- Creamed, creamy, in cream sauce
- Fried, deep-fried, french-fried, batter-fried, pan-fried
- Gravy, hollandaise, parmigiana, pastry, rich, sautéed, scalloped or escalloped, seasoned, Southern style

Look for these low-fat words instead:
- Baked, broiled, boiled, grilled, poached
- Roasted, steamed, stir-fried

*

Your Restaurant Options:

GO! Lower-fat choices	CAUTION! High-fat choices

Pizza

• Pizza without cheese • Onions, green peppers, mushrooms	• Meat toppings (sausage/pepperoni) • Olives

Burger Place (fast food)

• Grilled, broiled, or roasted chicken, without sauce • Broiled, extra-lean burger	• Regular hamburger, cheeseburger • French fries • Fried fish or chicken • Mayonnaise-based sauces

Mexican

• Heated (not fried) tortillas • Grilled chicken or beef fajitas • Soft tacos (corn or flour tortillas) • Salsa	• Enchiladas • Chili con queso • Fried tortillas, tortilla chips • Sour cream, guacamole • Crisp tacos

Chinese and Japanese

• Stir-fried chicken • Stir-fried vegetables • Steamed rice • Soup • Teriyaki	• Egg foo yong • Fried chicken, beef, or fish • Fried rice or noodles • Egg rolls • Fried wonton • Tempura

Italian

• Spaghetti with meatless tomato sauce • Minestrone soup	• Sausage • Lasagna, manicotti, other pasta dishes with cheese or cream • Fried or breaded dishes (like veal or eggplant parmigiana)

Seafood

• Broiled, baked, or boiled seafood with lemon • Plain baked potato	• Fried fish • Fried vegetables • French fries

Steak Houses

• Shrimp cocktail • Broiled chicken or fish • Plain baked potato	• Steak (except trimmed lean cuts) • Fried fish or chicken • Onion rings, other fried vegetables • French fries

green peas, kale, lima beans, potatoes, spinach, squash, sweet potatoes, and tomatoes (essentially all vegetables).

Typical serving sizes include: 1 cup of raw vegetables; ½ cup of cooked vegetables; ½ cup of vegetable juice.

Eat 4 to 5 Daily Servings of Fruits

The DASH diet has more daily servings of fresh fruits than many eating plans because fruits are such important sources of protective nutrients and fiber. Fruits are high in potassium, which helps keep blood pressure levels healthy. In fact, a potassium-rich diet may help to reduce elevated or high blood pressure, which is important for preventing or managing complications of diabetes. Examples of fruits are apples, apricots, bananas, dates, grapefruit, grapes, mangoes, melons, oranges, peaches, pineapples, raisins, strawberries, and tangerines.

Typical serving sizes include: 1 medium fruit; ¼ cup of dried fruit; 1 cup of chopped fresh fruit.

Eat 2 to 3 Daily Servings of Fat-free or Low-fat Milk and Milk Products

These foods are major sources of calcium and protein. Good-for-you choices include: fat-free (skim) or low-fat (1% milk) or buttermilk; fat-free, low-fat, or reduced-fat cheese; fat-free or low-fat yogurt. If you have trouble digesting milk and milk products, try taking lactase enzyme pills (available at drugstores and groceries) with the milk products. Or buy lactose-free milk, which has the lactase enzyme already added to it.

Typical serving sizes include: 1 cup of milk or yogurt; 1½ ounces of cheese.

Eat 6 or Fewer Daily Servings of Lean Meats, Poultry, and Fish

These foods are high in protein. Be sure to select only lean meats, and trim away all visible fat. Also, broil, roast, or poach these proteins to cut down on fat, and remove skin from poultry. Since eggs are high in cholesterol, limit your egg yolk consumption to no more than three per week; two egg whites have the same protein content as one ounce of meat.

Typical serving sizes include: 1 ounce of cooked meat, poultry, or fish; 1 egg (or 2 egg whites).

Eat Nuts, Seeds, and Legumes 4 to 5 Times Weekly

Rich sources of energy, these foods are high in magnesium, protein, and fiber—all nutrients that are important in controlling and managing diabetes. Examples include almonds, hazelnuts, kidney beans, lentils, mixed nuts, peanuts, split peas, sunflower seeds, and walnuts. These make much better snacks than packaged chips. If you are allergic to nuts, use seeds or legumes such as cooked dried beans or peas.

Typical serving sizes include: ⅓ cup or 1½ ounces of nuts; 2 tablespoons of peanut butter; 2 tablespoons or ½ ounce of seeds; ½ cup of cooked legumes.

Eat 2 to 3 Daily Servings of Fats and Oils

The DASH diet has roughly 27 percent of calories as fat, including fat in or added to foods. Good choices include soft margarine, vegetable oil (such as canola, corn, olive, safflower), low-fat mayonnaise, and light salad dressings.

Typical serving sizes include: 1 teaspoon of soft margarine; 1 teaspoon of vegetable oil; 1 tablespoon of mayonnaise; 2 tablespoons of salad dressing.

Reduce the Sodium in Your Diet

To eat a diet low in sodium, you need to do more than just avoid adding salt to your food. Here are some suggestions:

* Buy fresh, plain frozen, or canned vegetables without added salt.
* Choose ready-to-eat cereals that are lower in sodium.
* Use fresh poultry, fish, and lean meat instead of smoked or processed, such as hot dogs, ham, sausage, or luncheon meats.
* Avoid salty snack foods and crackers.

Both the DPP-based diet and the DASH diet outlined for you in this chapter will certainly help to improve your overall health and assist in preventing or managing your diabetes. They're low in fat and minimize processed foods. In many people, the symptoms of diabetes may diminish as a result of following these plans; in others, medication requirements could be adjusted downward or eliminated. Once you work either of these diets into your lifestyle, eating for prevention or management will become second nature—a

**Overview of DASH to Manage Diabetes—
How Much Do You Eat?**

Food Group	*Number of Daily Servings
Grains	6 to 8 servings
Vegetables	4 to 5 servings
Fruit	4 to 5 servings
Low-fat Dairy Products	2 to 3 servings
Lean Meats, Poultry, and Fish	6 or fewer servings
Nuts, Seeds, and Legumes	4 to 5 times weekly
Fats and Oils	2 to 3 servings

*If you need to lose weight, choose the serving size that is lower on the daily range.

habit that can enhance the quality of your health and your life. Along with these diets, there are some additional nutritional guidelines I'll discuss below that you can apply to further change your eating habits for the better.

Another Nutrition Tool: Carbohydrate Counting

Whether you follow the DPP or DASH-based recommendations, you may want to consider a tool called "carbohydrate counting." This is a method of controlling the amount of carbohydrates you eat at meals and snacks. The reason for counting carbohydrates is that they have the greatest impact on your blood sugar. If you know how much carbohydrate you've eaten, you can predict what your blood glucose will do, since the amount of carbohydrate you eat (whether sugar or starch) will determine how high your blood sugar level will be after a meal or snack.

For some people, carbohydrate counting is easier to learn than many other systems. The fact that it provides an accurate guess of how your blood sugar will rise after a meal or snack is of particular importance if you take insulin, which is required to balance your glucose levels. The amount of carbohydrate in a meal largely determines how many units of insulin you require. Counting carbohydrates, therefore, can help you make appropriate insulin adjustments based on your blood glucose patterns.

One caveat, however: Counting carbohydrates doesn't mean counting any type of carb. Continue to reach for whole grains, fruits, and vegetables—unprocessed foods—as your carbs of choice.

There are two methods of carbohydrate counting: simple and advanced. With the simple method, you work with your dietitian to plan how many grams of carbohydrate to eat at meals and snacks. One serving of bread, starches, fruit, or milk, for example, contains between 12 and 15 grams of carbohydrate. (Vegetables contribute little carbohydrate and are not counted.) When you know how many grams of carbohydrate you need at each meal, you can choose foods from any of the carbohydrate-containing food groups to meet your allowance. Knowing the carbohydrate amount in certain portions of food is important too. For instance, a medium-size baked potato is usually around 5 ounces and contains 35 grams of carbohydrate, while a large baked potato—the type you often get at restaurants—is about 7 or 8 ounces and has about 55 grams of carbohydrate.

The advanced method of carbohydrate counting is highly useful if you take short-acting insulin. This method matches your insulin dose to the amount of carbohydrate grams to be eaten. People who use this method usually take three to four insulin injections daily, or use an insulin pump. If you choose this method, you must understand how to use food labels, use measuring cups and spoons to measure your food portions, and be skilled at estimating carbohydrate content of restaurant foods. Keep records of your food intake and blood sugar, and use these records to determine the amount of insulin to take for the amount of carbohydrate you wish to eat. This is called a *carbohydrate to insulin ratio*. It's important to work with a professional diabetes team to help you determine your individual carbohydrate to insulin ratio.

In carbohydrate counting, the focus is on carbohydrates, but remember that lean proteins and good fats are still important. When protein and fat are eaten at the same time as carbohydrate, your blood sugar may not rise as quickly.

Weighing and Measuring Your Foods

Weighing and measuring food is extremely important in order to get the correct number of daily calories on either eating plan. As you begin your new diet, use measuring cups and spoons, and a food scale that measures ounces.

After measuring all foods for a week or so, you'll be able to make fairly accurate estimates by eye or by holding food without having to measure everything every time you eat. If you're dining out and can't measure, use the following visual references to help you gauge serving sizes:

- 1 cup of food is the size of a large handful, or 8 fluid ounces of liquid.
- ½ cup of food is about half of a large handful, or 4 fluid ounces of liquid.
- 1 tablespoon is about the size of the tip of your thumb (from the last joint crease).
- 1 teaspoon is about the size of the tip of your little finger (from the last joint crease).
- 3 to 4 ounces of cooked lean meat, fish, or poultry is about the size of a deck of cards.
- 1 ounce of hard cheese is about the size of a domino.
- A serving of vegetables is ½ cup (½ handful) cooked, or 1 cup (1 handful) raw.

What About Alcohol?

Some studies have suggested that light to moderate alcohol intake may have specific benefits for people with type 2 diabetes. Red wine, in particular, appears to have health benefits due to its high antioxidant content. Here is a good rule of thumb: when your diabetes is well-controlled, moderate use of alcohol—no more than two drinks per day for men and not more than one drink for women—generally may not affect your blood sugar. Even so, please follow these guidelines:

- Do not drink alcohol if you have been diagnosed with pancreatitis, abnormal blood fats, kidney disease, or nerve disease.
- Because alcohol may increase the risk of low blood sugar if you are using insulin or taking a sulfonylurea (a type of diabetes drug), have your alcoholic beverage with a meal if you have it at all.
- If you need to lose weight, do not drink alcohol, since alcoholic beverages are high in calories and promote weight gain.
- If you are pregnant or have a history of alcohol abuse, abstain from drinking alcohol altogether.

Artificial Sweeteners

It is fine to include artificial sweeteners in your diet, and sugar-free foods that contain them, as long as you go easy on these products. It's best to get used to the natural sweetness in fruits than rely on artificial sweeteners. But if you enjoy a sweet taste every now and then, there are several sweeteners on the market:

- Saccharin is found in Sugar Twin, Sweet'n Low, Sucaryl, and Featherweight. Some previous studies found that large amounts of saccharin cause bladder cancer in rats, but the rats were fed huge amounts that would not apply to human diets.
- Aspartame (NutraSweet and Equal) has come under scrutiny because of rare reports of neurologic disorders, including headaches or dizziness, associated with its use. It has been studied more intensively than any other food additive, however, and concern about any major health dangers is largely unfounded.
- Sucralose (Splenda) is made from table sugar and is six hundred times as sweet as sugar. It cannot be digested; therefore, it adds no calories. Several studies have shown that it does not affect blood glucose levels.
- Also known as acesulfame-K, acesulfame potassium (Sweet One and SwissSweet) is a calorie-free sweetener that has been used in foods and beverages around the world for fifteen years. The ingredient, which is two hundred times sweeter than sugar, has been used in numerous foods in the United States since 1988. In the United States, it is used in such products as candies, baked goods, frozen desserts, beverages, dessert mixes, and tabletop sweeteners. Acesulfame potassium is often used in combination with other low-calorie sweeteners because it enhances the sweet taste of foods and beverages.
- Found in many dietetic foods, sorbitol, mannitol, and xylitol are common sugar alcohols that produce a lower glycemic response than sugar and other carbohydrates. Although they offer no significant benefit, in large amounts, they may have a laxative effect.

Beware of "Diet" Foods

If you're trying to lose weight and get healthier, you may be surprised to find out that many diet foods—sugar-free, fat-free, and low-fat products—have the same number of calories as their nondiet counterparts—and they are highly processed. Many fat-free foods, for example, have as many calories as their full-fat counterparts. These calories come from fat replacers produced from starches or proteins. Check the nutrition labels. As much as possible, stick to natural, nonprocessed foods like lean meats, vegetables, whole grains, and fruits. Your body will thank you for it.

What about the Glycemic Index?

Some people today are concerned with the impact of the glycemic index on diabetes. The glycemic index, or GI, ranks carbohydrates based on how they affect your levels of blood sugar. High-GI foods, like cornflakes, potatoes, and white bread, greatly affect blood glucose levels. Low-GI foods, such as oatmeal, beans, sweet potatoes, nuts, and skim milk, produce less of an effect. Some recent weight-loss diets have included this popular concept of the glycemic index and have attempted to link low-GI foods to weight loss and high-GI foods to weight gain.

The glycemic index in the treatment of diabetes is and has been controversial since it was created twenty-five years ago. The new dietary guidelines from the American Diabetes Association provide no support for the use of the glycemic index in the management of diabetes. Some physicians endorse it, and others do not. While I do not necessarily support the glycemic index, it needs to be included in this book so that you may make your own decision as to its use in consultation with your physician.

The problem with the use of the glycemic index, and at the root of its controversy, is that the idea of classifying foods into groups—those that greatly affect your blood glucose and those that don't—is a very appealing concept to people with diabetes. But it's not quite that simple, and here's why:

* GI varies depending on the kind of food, how ripe it is, how long it was stored, how you cook it, the variety of the food (Australian potatoes have a higher GI than U.S. potatoes), and how the food may have been processed.

- GI varies among individuals and even in the same individual, depending on your blood glucose level, insulin resistance, and other factors.
- GI of a food may be different based on whether it is eaten alone or whether it is eaten with other foods as part of an entire meal.
- GI values are based on a 50-gram carbohydrate portion, not an amount typically eaten.
- Some foods with a low GI aren't necessarily healthy. For example, pizza, which is high in fat, has a low GI, and isn't a good option when eaten on a regular basis. High-fructose corn syrup, which also has a low GI, is linked to overweight and obesity.
- And finally, most GI values are based on blood glucose response to food for two hours, but glucose levels after eating some foods remain elevated for up to four hours or more in diabetics.

So, now you understand the controversy.

Again, if you still desire to give the glycemic index a try, there are a number of books that can guide you in this direction and a number of resources to locate the GI of common foods. Remember, however, that you may not be able to find the GI of every food you would potentially consume.

Avoid Popular Diets

Some fad diets skimp on nutrients and can be harmful in the long run. I recommend that you stay away from these diets if you are trying to prevent diabetes, manage it, or lose weight. Refer to the chart on the following page to review comparison among various diets.

Using Meal Replacements to Control Your Weight

Worth mentioning is a follow-up study to the Diabetes Prevention Program called Look AHEAD (Action for Health in Diabetes). This program recruited people with type 2 diabetes and used a lifestyle strategy similar to the DPP. Because of the need to promote a fairly rapid weight loss in the participants, this study used meal replacements and for this reason I present this option.

Calorie-controlled meal replacements are liquid formulas or packaged

Type of Diet	Fat, as % of Calories	Nutritional Profile
High-fat, Low-carbohydrate Diets Examples: Atkins Diet South Beach Diet Zone Diet Sugar Busters Protein Power	Greater than 50% of calories from fat	Low in several nutrients: vitamins A, B_6, D, and E, thiamine, folate, calcium, magnesium, iron, zinc, potassium, and dietary fiber. Contains excess amounts of total fat, saturated fat, and dietary cholesterol. Supplements are highly recommended when one is on a low-calorie, high-fat diet.
Moderate-fat Diets Examples: DASH Diet American Diabetic Association Weight Watchers Jenny Craig Sonoma Diet	25% to 30% of calories from fat	Usually, a nutritionally balanced eating plan assuming you eat a variety of foods from all categories. However, limiting certain food categories can lead to deficiencies in nutrients, especially calcium, zinc, and iron.

Low-fat and Very Low-fat Diets
Volumetrics
Dean Ornish's Eat
  More, Weigh Less
New Pritikin
  Program
	10% to 20% of calories from fat	Can be deficient in zinc and vitamin B_{12} because of infrequent meat consumption. Can be inadequate in vitamin E, a fat-soluble vitamin found in oils, nuts, and other foods rich in fat.

items with a fixed number of calories. Their use in weight control not only works, according to a number of studies, but also makes absolute sense. Using a meal replacement to stand in for a meal takes the guesswork out of meal planning. By controlling portion sizes, fat, and carbohydrate, you can control calories. Meal replacements are generally balanced and contain a mix of protein, carbohydrate, and fat, as well as other nutrients. Four different types of meal replacements are available: powder mixes, shakes, bars, and prepackaged meals, such as frozen dinners. The usual plan is to use a meal replacement for one or two meals a day while having sensible meals that combine lean meat with whole, natural, complex carbohydrates, vegetables, and fruit for the other meals during the day. A meal replacement plan is provided on page 89 as a guide to assisting you in your weight control efforts.

Manage Stress

It's natural that when you make any type of lifestyle change, there can be stress associated with it. And often, that stress can trigger overeating or inactivity. But you do not have to let stress derail your efforts or make you feel out of control. Here are some strategies to help you manage the potential stress of changing your diet and lifestyle:

A Meal Replacement Plan for Weight Loss	
Breakfast	A meal replacement
Lunch	A meal replacement or sensible meal of protein, carbohydrate, vegetables, and fruit
Dinner	A sensible meal of protein, carbohydrate, vegetables, and fruit
Snack	Fruit, vegetables, fat-free yogurt or cheese, nuts, or air-popped popcorn

Staying on Track

I don't expect you to stick to your diabetes prevention or management 100 percent of the time. You may have a slip every now and then—times when you don't follow your plans for healthy eating or being active. These are a normal part of lifestyle change and are to be expected. They don't hurt your progress. What hurts your progress is the way you *react* to slips. You don't want to get upset, or beat yourself up for not sticking 100 percent to your program. That's self-defeating and only sets you up for more of the same. Try to learn from your slip. Ask yourself: what caused you to slip from healthy eating or exercising? Can you avoid it in the future? Manage it better? You are making lifelong changes, and slips are just one part of the process. In the chart on the following page are some ways to stay on track.

In the next chapter, I offer menus and recipes that are appropriate if you have diabetes, or hope to prevent it. Based on the DPP and the DASH recommendations, they include many of the concepts presented in this chapter and are designed to help you begin to live better and feel more healthy.

Possible source of stress	Ways to manage stress	Examples
Extra time spent in food preparation, shopping	• Share some of your work. • Take charge of your time.	• Ask your spouse to help you shop. • Make double recipes. Freeze part for later.
Feel deprived when can't eat favorite foods	• Set goals you can reach. • Keep things in perspective.	• Allow yourself to have favorite foods in small amounts now and then. • Remind yourself how important preventing diabetes is to you.
Upset if your family doesn't like low-fat foods	• Reach out to people. • Use the steps for solving problems.	• Ask your family to support your efforts to try new foods. • Discuss your feelings and your commitment to weight loss with your family. Brainstorm options with them. Try one.
Feel uncomfortable participating in social activities where high-fat foods are available	• Practice saying no. • Reach out to people. • Plan ahead.	• Turn down invitations that aren't important to you. • Call the host or hostess ahead and ask what will be served and if you can bring a low-fat dish. • Before you go to a party, plan what foods you will choose.
Feel stressed by trying to fit activity into an already busy schedule	• Plan ahead. • Problem solve.	• Make an appointment to be active. • Combine activity with other events you plan to do anyhow. (Take a walking meeting. Go hiking with the family.)

Ways to Stay Motivated

1. Stay aware of the benefits you've achieved and hope to achieve.

2. Recognize your successes.
   What changes in your eating and activity do you feel most proud?

3. Keep visible signs of your progress.
   Post weight and activity graphs on your refrigerator door.
   Mark your activity milestones on a map toward a particular goal.
   Measure yourself (waist, belt size) once a month.

4. Keep track of your weight, eating, and activity.
   Record your activity daily.
   Record what you eat.
   Record your weight regularly.

(continued)

Ways to Stay Motivated
(continued)

5. Add variety to your routine.
   How have you varied your activity?
   What meals, snacks, or foods are you most bored with?
   Can you think of some ways to vary this part of your eating?

6. Set new goals for yourself and reward yourself when you meet each goal.
   Goals: specific, short-term, just enough of a challenge.
   Rewards: something you will do or buy *if and only if* you reach your goal.
   What are some nonfood ways you can reward yourself for reaching a goal?

7. Create some friendly competition.
   Set up the kind of competition in which you both win.

8. Use friends, family, and others to help you stay motivated.
   Call them for encouragement and support.

ASK DR. CEFALU: DOES DIABETES AFFECT MY DIGESTION?

If you have diabetic-related nerve damage, you may experience gastropare-sis, in which the stomach takes too long to empty itself. It may occur in people with either type 1 or type 2 diabetes. Symptoms of gastroparesis include heartburn, nausea, vomiting of undigested food, an early feeling of fullness when eating, and abdominal bloating. To treat gastroparesis, your doctor will advise that you eat smaller, more frequent meals and may prescribe med-ications to stimulate stomach contractions.

＊

ASK DR. CEFALU: I'M OVERWEIGHT. HOW DOES THIS AFFECT THE
LIKELIHOOD THAT I MIGHT DEVELOP DIABETES?

Being overweight or obese is a leading risk factor for type 2 diabetes be-cause the extra pounds make it difficult for cells to respond to insulin, a condition called insulin resistance. Often, people with type 2 diabetes are able to lower their blood glucose by losing weight and increasing their exer-cise. Dropping pounds also helps lower the risk for other health problems that especially affect people with diabetes, such as cardiovascular disease. If you lose a mere 5 to 7 percent of your body weight, you can delay, and possi-bly prevent, type 2 diabetes.

＊

5

Meal Plans and Recipes to Prevent or Manage Diabetes

FOOD IS CLEARLY A POWERFUL TOOL IN the treatment of prediabetes and diabetes and plays a huge role in preventing and managing the disease. This chapter practically applies the guidelines of the previous chapter by giving six weeks' worth of menus that would generally fit into the DPP or DASH regimens, as described in Chapter 4. These easy-to-follow menus include tasty meal options (with recipes), as well as snacks. Your nutrients have been tallied for the entire day, so you don't have to do any counting. All of the menus are low in fat, high in fiber, packed with nutrition, and provide calories in a range from 1,100 to 1,400 calories a day for steady weight loss. Throughout the chapter, special features are included to help you save time and get healthy, including ideas for quick meals; strategies for business lunches; and travel and vacations. Here are some additional guidelines:

- A total of forty-two menu plans will give you many options—forty-two days or more if you wish.
- These diets are designed in appropriate calorie ranges for weight loss. However, if you need more calories daily, add those in from extra fruit or vegetable servings each day, or from a few more ounces of protein (unless your physician has instructed you to restrict your protein intake).
- You may change the order of the menus or use the same breakfasts, lunches, dinners, or snacks you like as often as you wish. Also, any fruits, vegetables, protein, or dairy foods that are specified in the meal plan may be substituted with others in the same food group, if you prefer. If you dislike fish, for example, substitute a different protein. To save more fat, choose lower-fat versions of foods listed, if available.
- Drink fluids, preferably water, throughout the day. Most people require about eight cups of fresh water daily for good health. It's fine to enjoy herbal teas, as well as coffee and diet soft drinks, but do so in moderation.

This new dietary lifestyle, if followed faithfully, will become a second-nature habit—one that will lead to much-improved health and a greater quality of life.

Starred items (*) have a recipe, found at the end of the chapter.

* Day 1 *

BREAKFAST	LUNCH	DINNER	SNACK
* Raspberry Smoothie	1 serving meatless chili; 1 apple	3 ounces grilled salmon; ½ cup cooked brown rice; 1 cup steamed spinach; 1 cup sliced fresh peaches	1 ounce cheddar cheese with 4 whole wheat crackers

Nutrition information: 1,205 calories, 85 grams protein, 152 grams carbohydrate, 35 grams fat, 30 grams fiber

* Day 2 *

BREAKFAST	LUNCH	DINNER	SNACK
1 cup skim or low-fat milk; 1 serving high-fiber cereal; 1 cup blueberries	*Shrimp and Rice Salad	3 ounces baked chicken; 1 medium baked sweet potato; 1 cup steamed broccoli or other vegetable; tossed salad with 2 table-spoons low-fat dressing; 1 apple, baked, sprinkled with cinnamon	1 fresh pear, sliced, with 1 cup low-fat, sugar-free yogurt

Nutrition information: 1,176 calories, 82 grams protein, 202 grams carbohydrate, 12 grams fat, 34 grams fiber

* Day 3 *

BREAKFAST	LUNCH	DINNER	SNACK
2 scrambled egg whites, or 1 serving egg substitute; *Oat Bran Muffin; ½ cup grapefruit sections	3 ounces grilled chicken breast; *Baked Sweet Potato Fries; tossed salad with 2 table-spoons low-fat dressing; 1 cup fresh pineapple chunks	*Two-Minute Burritos with *Avocado and Tomato Salsa	*Strawberries in Balsamic Vinegar with 1 cup low-fat, sugar-free yogurt

Nutrition information: 1,280 calories, 66 grams protein, 218 grams carbohydrate, 22 grams fat, 41 grams fiber

* Day 4 *

BREAKFAST	LUNCH	DINNER	SNACK
*Oatmeal with Fruit	*Black Bean Soup; tossed salad with 2 tablespoons low-fat dressing; 1 apple	3 ounces lean grilled steak; 1 cup steamed Brussels sprouts;1 medium baked potato	1 cup fresh straw-berries with 1 cup low-fat, sugar-free yogurt

Nutrition information: 1,292 calories, 83 grams protein, 224 grams carbohydrate, 14 grams fat, 37 grams fiber

* Day 5 *

BREAKFAST	LUNCH	DINNER	SNACK
½ cup low-fat cottage cheese; ½ cup fresh pineapple chunks; 1 slice rye toast	*Salmon and Vegetable Salad; 1 orange	3 ounces baked turkey; 1 cup steamed carrots; 1 cup steamed, mashed cauliflower	1 apple; 2 ounces cheddar cheese

Nutrition information: 1,100 calories, 65 grams protein, 150 grams carbohydrate, 29 grams fat, 32 grams fiber

* Day 6 *

BREAKFAST	LUNCH	DINNER	SNACK
1 cup low-fat, sugar-free yogurt; ½ cup low-fat granola; 1 cup berries	Deli-type sandwich: 1 slice low-fat turkey, 1 slice low-fat cheese, lettuce and tomato, 1 teaspoon yellow mustard	3 ounces grilled chicken; 1 cup steamed summer squash; tossed salad with low-fat dressing; 1 cup fresh melon balls	*Apple Smoothie

Nutrition information: 1,100 calories, 72 grams protein, 180 grams carbohydrate, 13 grams fat, 27 grams fiber

* Day 7 *

BRUNCH	DINNER	SNACK
*Potato Kale Frittata; ⅛ cantaloupe	Grilled tuna steak; *Sautéed Broccoli and Garlic; 1 cup cooked brown rice	1 cup low-fat, sugar-free vanilla yogurt with 1 banana, sliced

Nutrition information: 1,100 calories, 52 grams protein, 145 grams carbohydrate, 25 grams fat, 16 grams fiber

* Day 8 *

BREAKFAST	LUNCH	DINNER	SNACK
*Oat Bran Bread French Toast, topped with ½ cup sliced baked apples	*Creamy Broccoli Soup; 1 orange	Lean grilled steak; 1 medium baked potato; tossed salad with 2 tablespoons low-fat dressing	1 apple; 6 almonds or walnuts

Nutrition information: 1,140 calories, 51 grams protein, 160 grams carbohydrate, 35 grams fat, 27 grams fiber

BREAKFAST	LUNCH	DINNER	SNACK
*Tofu Colada	Tuna salad sandwich (3 ounces water-packed tuna with 1 tablespoon low-fat mayonnaise) in a whole wheat pita, 1 raw carrot	*Bell Pepper Lasagna; tossed salad with 1 table-spoon low-fat dressing	1 banana; 1 cup soy milk

Nutrition information: 1,100 calories, 62 grams protein, 152 grams carbohydrate, 21 grams fat, and 18 grams fiber

BREAKFAST	LUNCH	DINNER	SNACK
1 scrambled egg; 1 slice multigrain toast; 1 cup fresh blueberries	*Chicken Wild Rice Salad with Mango	3 ounces roasted pork tenderloin; *Braised Red Cabbage with Apple	1 cup low-fat, sugar-free yogurt; 1 fresh plum

Nutrition information: 1,133 calories, 81 grams protein, 111 grams carbohydrate, 39 grams fat, 14 grams fiber

BREAKFAST	LUNCH	DINNER	SNACK
½ whole wheat bagel with 1 table-spoon nonfat cream cheese; *Broiled Grapefruit; 1 cup low-fat, sugar-free yogurt	*Tuna Nicoise Salad; 1 apple	*Beefsteak with Tomato-Orange Salsa	*Eggplant Dip (¼ cup) with fresh chopped vegetables

Nutrition information: 1,100 calories, 80 grams protein, 159 grams carbohydrate, 12 grams fat, 25 grams fiber

* Day 12 *

BREAKFAST	LUNCH	DINNER	SNACK
1 poached egg; ½ whole wheat English muffin, toasted; 1 cup fresh raspberries	*Butternut Squash and Orange Soup; 4 wheat crackers; tossed salad with 2 tablespoons reduced-fat French dressing; 1 cup chopped fresh pineapple	*Fish in Spicy Tomato Sauce; ½ cup cooked brown rice; 1 cup steamed green beans	1 cup low-fat, sugar-free vanilla yogurt; 1 cup fresh strawberries

Nutrition information: 1,100 calories, 51 grams protein, 176 grams carbohydrate, 24 grams fat, 31 grams fiber

* Day 13 *

BREAKFAST	LUNCH	DINNER	SNACK
½ cup high-fiber bran cereal; 1 cup soy milk; 1 cup fresh strawberries	Spinach salad: 2 cups chopped fresh spinach, 1 large slice of onion, 2 ounces feta cheese, 2 tablespoons fat-free cranberry or raspberry balsamic vinaigrette dressing; 1 fresh peach	2 slices extra-lean ham; 1 medium sweet potato, baked in skin; 1 cup boiled cabbage; 1 baked apple, sprinkled with cinnamon	1 cup low-fat, sugar-free yogurt and 1 banana, sliced

Nutrition information: 1,200 calories, 60 grams protein, 201 grams carbohydrate, 25 grams fat, 34 grams fiber

* Day 14 *

BREAKFAST	LUNCH	DINNER	SNACK
*Strawberry-Orange Smoothie; 1 slice whole-grain toast	⅛ of a 12" pizza, meat and vegetable topping, regular crust; tossed salad with 1 tablespoon reduced-fat dressing; 1 apple	3 ounces Alaskan King crab, steamed; 1 ear of corn; 1 cup coleslaw; 1 cup low-fat, sugar-free yogurt	2 ounces cheddar cheese; 4 wheat crackers

Nutrition information: 1,300 calories, 65 grams protein, 167 grams carbohydrate, 45 grams fat, 22 grams fiber

BREAKFAST	LUNCH	DINNER	SNACK
1 scrambled or poached egg; 1 cup raisin bran cereal; 1 cup low-fat, 1% milk; ½ fresh grapefruit	Sandwich: 6 thin slices smoked turkey breast, 2 slices reduced-calorie bread, 1 teaspoon yellow mustard, sliced tomato and lettuce; 1 fresh plum	3 ounces grilled or baked salmon, cooked; ½ cup cooked long-grain rice; 1 cup steamed summer squash; 1 cup low-fat, sugar-free yogurt	1 apple; 1 cup soy milk

Nutrition information: 1,400 calories, 75 grams protein, 231 grams carbohydrate, 26 grams fat, 30 grams fiber

BREAKFAST	LUNCH	DINNER	SNACK
1 cup low-fat, sugar-free yogurt; 1 orange; ½ cup cooked oat bran; 1 cup skim milk	1 cup meatless chili; tossed salad with 2 tablespoons reduced-fat dressing; 1 apple	3 ounces grilled boneless, skinless chicken breast; ½ cup cooked lima beans; 1 cup steamed cauliflower	1 cup low-fat, sugar-free yogurt; 1 piece fresh fruit

Nutrition information: 1,200 calories, 88 grams protein, 179 grams carbohydrate, 18 grams fat, 30 grams fiber

BREAKFAST	LUNCH	DINNER	SNACK
1 hard-boiled egg; 1 cup Special K cereal; 1 cup soy milk; 1 cup fresh strawberries	Tuna salad: 3 ounces drained, water-packed light tuna, 1 cup chopped romaine lettuce, 1 cup chopped raw tomatoes, 2 tablespoons bottled balsamic vinaigrette dressing; ½ cup cooked brown rice; 1 orange	3 ounces broiled beef, top sirloin; sweet potato, baked in skin; 1 cup steamed green beans	1 fresh kiwifruit, sliced

Nutrition information: 1,126 calories, 74 grams protein, 165 grams carbohydrate, 22 grams fat, 26 grams fiber

* Day 18 *

BREAKFAST	LUNCH	DINNER	SNACK
2 slices cooked turkey bacon; *Oat Bran Muffin; 1 cup tomato juice	1 flour tortilla with beef filling; 1 side salad (lettuce and salad vegetables) with 1 tablespoon reduced-fat dressing; 1 apple	3 ounces baked Cornish game hen, skin removed; ½ cup cooked long-grain rice; 1 cup steamed Brussels sprouts with 1 tea-spoon trans fat–free margarine	1 fresh pear

Nutrition information: 1,112 calories, 51 grams protein, 178 grams carbohydrate, 20 grams fat, 20 grams fiber

* Day 19 *

BREAKFAST	LUNCH	DINNER	SNACK
2 reduced-fat sausage links; ½ cup oatmeal (regular); 1 cup low-fat, 1% milk; 1 cup fresh blueberries	1 grilled lean hamburger patty; 1 tomato, sliced; side salad with 1 tablespoon reduced-fat Italian salad dressing	3 ounces grilled or baked white fish; 1 cup steamed spinach; ½ cup sweet corn; 10 fresh cherries	1 cup low-fat, sugar-free yogurt

Nutrition information: 1,159 calories, 76 grams protein, 172 grams carbohydrate, 25 grams fat, 20 grams fiber

* Day 20 *

BREAKFAST	LUNCH	DINNER	SNACK
½ cup low-fat cottage cheese; 1 cup fresh rasp-berries; 1 slice oatmeal bread, toasted	3 ounces cooked turkey breast, skin removed; 1 slice *each* fresh tomato and onion with 1 tablespoon balsamic vinaigrette dressing; 1 slice stone-ground whole wheat bread; 1 orange	3 ounces shrimp, steamed; ½ cup cooked brown rice; 1 cup boiled cabbage; 1 apple	1 cup fresh strawberries

Nutrition information: 1,100 calories, 60 grams protein, 164 grams carbohydrate, 21 grams fat, 21 grams fiber

* Day 21 *

BREAKFAST	LUNCH	DINNER	SNACK
1 scrambled or poached egg; ½ cup high-fiber bran cereal; 1 cup low-fat, 1% milk; 1 cup fresh strawberries	1 cup vegetable soup; 1 ounce cheddar cheese; 4 whole wheat crackers; 1 fresh pear	*Shepherd's Pie with Sweet Potato Topping; 1 cup chopped fresh fruit	3 cups air-popped popcorn

Nutrition information: 1,300 calories, 65 grams protein, 185 grams carbohydrate, 31 grams fat, 32 grams fiber

* Day 22 *

BREAKFAST	LUNCH	DINNER	SNACK
*Raspberry Smoothie	1 serving meatless chili; tossed salad with 2 tablespoons reduced-fat dressing; 1 apple	3 ounces grilled salmon; 1 cup cooked brown rice; 1 cup steamed broccoli; 1 cup sliced fresh peaches	*Eggplant Dip (¼ cup) with sliced cucumbers

Nutrition information: 1,157 calories, 72 grams protein, 181 grams carbohydrate, 17 grams fat, 37 grams fiber

* Day 23 *

BREAKFAST	LUNCH	DINNER	SNACK
1 poached egg on stone-ground whole wheat bread; 1 cup skim or low-fat milk; 1 cup fresh blackberries	*Shrimp and Rice Salad	3 ounces baked chicken; 1 medium baked sweet potato; 1 cup steamed broccoli or other vegetable; 1 apple, baked, sprinkled with cinnamon	1 cup fresh pineapple; 1 diabetic shake

Nutrition information: 1,262 calories, 85 grams protein, 201 grams carbohydrate, 17 grams fat, 33 grams fiber

* Day 24 *

BREAKFAST	LUNCH	DINNER	SNACK
2 scrambled egg whites or 1 serving egg substitute; *Oat Bran Muffin; ½ cup grapefruit sections; 1 cup soy milk	3 ounces grilled chicken breast; *Baked Sweet Potato Fries; tossed salad with 1 table-spoon low-fat dressing; 1 fresh pear	*Oven "Fried" Fish; 1 cup steamed summer squash; 1 orange	1 cup low-fat, sugar-free yogurt; ½ banana, sliced

Nutrition information: 1,317 calories, 92 grams protein, 204 grams carbohydrate, 19 grams fat, 31 grams fiber

* Day 25 *

BREAKFAST	LUNCH	DINNER	SNACK
½ cup oat bran; 1 cup skim, soy, or low-fat milk; *Broiled Grapefruit	*Black Bean Soup; tossed salad with 2 tablespoons low-fat dressing; 1 apple	Lean grilled steak; 1 cup steamed cauliflower; 1 medium baked sweet potato	1 cup low-fat, sugar-free yogurt; 6 almonds

Nutrition information: 1,168 calories, 79 grams protein, 193 grams carbohydrate, 14 grams fat, 37 grams fiber

* Day 26 *

BREAKFAST	LUNCH	DINNER	SNACK
½ cup low-fat cottage cheese; 1 cup fresh pine-apple chunks; 1 slice pumpernickel toast	*Salmon and Vege-table Salad; 1 cup fresh blueberries	3 ounces baked turkey; 1 cup cooked lima beans; 1 cup steamed green beans	*Rice Pudding

Nutrition information: 1,434 calories, 74 grams protein, 253 grams carbohydrate, 31 grams fat, 39 grams fiber

* Day 27 *

BREAKFAST	LUNCH	DINNER	SNACK
2 slices cooked turkey bacon; 1 cup low-fat, sugar-free yogurt; ½ cup low-fat granola; 1 cup fresh strawberries	*Curried Garbanzo Beans; tossed salad with 2 tablespoons reduced-fat dressing	3 ounces grilled chicken; ½ cup couscous; 1 cup steamed broccoli; 1 cup chopped fresh fruit	1 fresh apple

Nutrition information: 1,225 calories, 68 grams protein, 204 grams carbohydrate, 26 grams fat, 24 grams fiber

* Day 28 *

BREAKFAST	LUNCH	DINNER	SNACK
2 scrambled egg whites; *Oat Bran Muffin; orange	*Creamy Broccoli Soup; 1 slice rye bread, 1 apple	4 ounces lean grilled steak; 1 medium baked potato; tossed salad with 2 tablespoons low-fat dressing	*Sweet Potato Custard

Nutrition information: 1,131 calories, 56 grams protein, 187 grams carbohydrate, 25 grams fat, 28 grams fiber

* Day 29 *

BREAKFAST	LUNCH	DINNER	SNACK
1 cup raisin bran cereal; 1 cup low-fat, 1% milk; ½ fresh grapefruit	Sandwich: 6 thin slices smoked reduced-fat turkey breast, 2 slices pumpernickel bread, 1 teaspoon yellow mustard, with sliced tomatoes; 1 cup sliced fresh peaches	3 ounces salmon, sockeye, cooked, dry heat; 1 cup cooked brown rice; 1 cup steamed broccoli; 1 small whole wheat dinner roll; 1 cup low-fat, sugar-free yogurt	1 cup chopped fresh fruit

Nutrition information: 1,400 calories, 75 grams protein, 231 grams carbohydrate, 26 grams fat, 30 grams fiber

* Day 30 *

BREAKFAST	LUNCH	DINNER	SNACK
1 whole egg, scrambled; 1 cup fresh blueberries; 1 slice cracked-wheat toast	1 cup meatless chili; 1 cup coleslaw	3 ounces grilled skinless chicken breast; 1 ear yellow corn; 1 medium baked potato; 1 cup steamed green beans	1 cup low-fat, sugar-free yogurt

Nutrition information: 1,200 calories, 88 grams protein, 179 grams carbohydrate, 18 grams fat, 30 grams fiber

* Day 31 *

BREAKFAST	LUNCH	DINNER	SNACK
½ cup oatmeal with 1 cup fresh straw-berries; 1 cup low-fat milk	Tuna salad: 3 ounces drained, water-packed light tuna; 1 cup chopped romaine lettuce, 1 cup chopped raw tomato, 2 table-spoons bottled balsamic vinaigrette dressing; 1 medium orange	3 ounces broiled beef, top sirloin; sweet potato, baked in skin; 1 cup cooked peas; 1 fresh kiwifruit, sliced	1 cup low-fat soy milk

Nutrition information: 1,126 calories, 74 grams protein, 165 grams carbohydrate, 22 grams fat, 26 grams fiber

* Day 32 *

BREAKFAST	LUNCH	DINNER	SNACK
2 slices cooked tur-key bacon; 1 English muffin, toasted; 1 cup tomato juice	⅛ of a 12" pizza, meat and vegetable topping, regular crust;1 side salad (lettuce and salad vegetables) with 1 tablespoon reduced-fat dressing; 1 apple	1 cup beef stew; 1 piece *Scallion Corn Bread; ⅛ can-taloupe; 1 cup low-fat, 1% milk	1 cup kefir (cultured milk) smoothie (low-fat, strawberry banana)

*Nutrition information:*1,358 calories, 67 grams protein, 194 grams carbohydrate, 44 grams fat, 18 grams fiber

* Day 33 *

BREAKFAST	LUNCH	DINNER	SNACK
½ cup oatmeal (regular); 1 cup low-fat, 1% milk; 1 cup fresh blueberries	3 ounces grilled chicken breast; ½ cup cooked brown rice; side salad with 1 tablespoon reduced-fat Italian dressing	*Baked Tuna Steaks with Peppers and Mushrooms; 1 medium baked potato; 20 fresh cherries	1 cup low-fat, sugar-free yogurt

Nutrition information: 1,100 calories, 67 grams protein, 153 grams carbohydrate, 24 grams fat, 19 grams fiber

* Day 34 *

BREAKFAST	LUNCH	DINNER	SNACK
1 cup low-fat, sugar-free yogurt; 1 cup fresh raspberries; 1 slice oatmeal bread, toasted	Fast-food lunch:* 6-inch turkey breast sub with lettuce and vegetables (no dressing)	3 ounces Alaskan King crab, steamed; 1 ear of corn; 1 cup coleslaw; 1 piece *Scallion Corn Bread	1 cup sliced fresh peaches

Nutrition information: 1,100 calories, 60 grams protein, 164 grams carbohydrate, 21 grams fat, 21 grams fiber

* Day 35 *

BREAKFAST	LUNCH	DINNER	SNACK
½ cup high-fiber bran cereal; 1 cup low-fat, 1% milk; 1 cup fresh strawberries	1 cup vegetable soup; 1 ounce cheddar cheese; 4 whole wheat crackers; 1 fresh pear	3 ounces cooked beef, top sirloin; 1 medium baked potato; 1 dinner roll; 12 spears of steamed asparagus	1 cup low-fat, sugar-free yogurt

Nutrition information: 1,200 calories, 74 grams protein, 176 grams carbohydrate, 28 grams fat, 27 grams fiber

Nutrition information is approximate, since calorie and nutrient counts vary from restaurant to restaurant.

* Day 36 *

BREAKFAST	LUNCH	DINNER	SNACK
*Oat Bran Bread French Toast; 1 cup unsweetened applesauce	1 soft taco with beef filling; side salad with lettuce and salad vegetables with 2 tablespoons reduced-fat French dressing; 1 cup low-fat, 1% milk	3 ounces salmon, cooked; 1 cup cooked carrots; 1 cup mashed potatoes; 1 cup sliced fresh peaches	2 dried figs

Nutrition information: 1,200 calories, 54 grams protein, 182 grams carbohydrate, 31 grams fat, 20 grams fiber

* Day 37 *

BREAKFAST	LUNCH	DINNER	SNACK
1 poached egg on an English muffin; ½ grapefruit; 1 cup soy milk	Caesar chicken salad with 2 table-spoons Caesar salad dressing; 1 bread stick; 1 cup fresh strawberries	2 slices extra-lean ham; 1 medium sweet potato, baked in skin; 1 cup boiled cabbage; 1 whole wheat dinner roll	1 cup low-fat, sugar-free yogurt

Nutrition information: 1,440 calories, 104 grams protein, 170 grams carbohydrate, 41 grams fat, 23 grams fiber

* Day 38 *

BREAKFAST	LUNCH	DINNER	SNACK
*Oat Bran Muffin; 1 cup fresh strawberries	Swiss cheese sandwich: 2 ounces Swiss cheese, 2 slices whole wheat bread, 1 teaspoon yellow mustard; sliced green pepper; 1 apple	1 cup cooked spaghetti with meat sauce; tossed salad with lettuce and salad vegeta-bles with 2 table-spoons reduced-fat Italian dressing; 1 cup low-fat, 1% milk	1 cup chopped fresh fruit

Nutrition information: 1,300 calories, 57 grams protein, 165 grams carbohydrate, 40 grams fat, 23 grams fiber

BREAKFAST	LUNCH	DINNER	SNACK
1 scrambled egg, 1 slice cracked-wheat toast, 1 fresh orange	*Black Bean Soup; 4 whole wheat crackers	Asian restaurant:* 1 cup beef with broccoli; 1 cup Chinese noodles; 1 cup chopped fresh pineapple; 1 cup 1% milk	3 cups air-popped popcorn

Nutrition information: 1,200 calories, 50 grams protein, 169 grams carbohydrate, 40 grams fat, 22 grams fiber

BREAKFAST	LUNCH	DINNER	SNACK
1 cup low-fat, sugar-free yogurt; 1 slice oatmeal bread, toasted	Pita sandwich: pita pocket, 6 table-spoons hummus, 1 peeled and thinly sliced cucumber; 1 cup soy milk	3 ounces grilled salmon; 1 cup cooked brown rice; 1 cup steamed chopped broccoli; 1 cup sliced fresh peaches	1 cup low-sodium vegetable juice; 1 raw carrot

Nutrition information: 1,137 calories, 58 grams protein, 173 grams carbohydrate, 25 grams fat, 23 grams fiber

BREAKFAST	LUNCH	DINNER	SNACK
1 cup low-fat, sugar-free, plain yogurt; 1 cup fresh blueberries; 1 slice oatmeal bread, toasted	Lunch at a restaurant:* grilled chicken sandwich (regular bun) with lettuce and tomato (no dressing)	3 ounces roasted pork loin; 1 cup applesauce; 1 cup steamed or boiled Brussels sprouts; 1 cup boiled carrots; 1 cup low-fat, sugar-free yogurt	1 granola bar

Nutrition information: 1,262 calories, 80 grams protein, 176 grams carbohydrate, 32 grams fat, 21 grams fiber

Nutrition information is approximate, since calorie and nutrient counts vary from restaurant to restaurant.

* Day 42 *

BREAKFAST	LUNCH	DINNER	SNACK
½ cup high-fiber bran cereal; 1 cup low-fat, 1% milk; 1 cup fresh raspberries	Spinach salad: 2 cups chopped fresh spinach, 1 large slice of onion, 2 ounces feta cheese, 2 table-spoons fat-free cranberry or rasp-berry balsamic vinaigrette dressing; 1 bread stick	*Chicken parmi-giana; ½ cup cooked whole wheat pasta; 1 cup steamed summer squash	1 cup chopped fresh fruit

Nutrition information: 1,210 calories, 71 grams protein, 189 grams carbohydrate, 24 grams fat, 27 grams fiber

---

IDEAS FOR QUICK AND EASY MEALS

- Once or twice a week, cut up salad ingredients and place them in covered plastic containers or plastic food-storage bags designed for vegetables. With the prep out of the way, simply toss veggies into a bowl and add left-over meats or seafood for a near-instant meal.
- Use labor-saving cooking devices. Add soup or stew ingredients to a slow cooker in the morning to simmer while you're at work. Pressure cookers are another way to cook meals quickly.
- Pair foods that can cook in the same pan or at the same oven temperature.
- Plan for more than one meal by cooking enough leftovers to make salads, soups, and stews.
- Pick up healthy, full-course meals at a supermarket that offers a large-scale deli and salad bar.
- Cook items like chicken breasts and brown rice in advance to save time. Stored properly, these items can keep for several days until you need them.
- Use meal replacement bars and shakes when you're in a hurry. Team them up with a piece of fresh fruit for a filling meal.

*

STRATEGIES FOR BUSINESS LUNCHES

- If you eat out on a regular basis, look for a way to bulk up your fiber intake with things like fresh fruit (especially berries), whole grains, and vegetable soups.
- Make a list of the restaurants and fast-food places that have the healthiest options (salads, soft-shell tacos, chili, or turkey subs are all great high-protein options).
- Brown-bag it when you can. For sandwiches, try hard-cooked eggs chopped and mixed with reduced-fat mayonnaise or reduced-fat salad dressing. Spice this up with chopped onion, celery, green pepper, or bean sprouts. Chop up leftover chicken and mix with reduced-fat mayonnaise or reduced-fat salad dressing and shredded raw vegetables. You can do the same with water-packed tuna.
- Be salad savvy at business lunches. Heap on fresh greens, beans, and veggies from the salad bar, but don't douse it with fatty dressings or high-fat toppings like cheese, eggs, bacon, or croutons. Instead, pick calorie-friendly vinaigrettes, low-fat dressings, even a generous squeeze of fresh lemon and ask for dressing on the side so that you can control the amount you eat.
- Watch out for potato salads, macaroni salads, coleslaw, even tuna and chicken salads, which usually are loaded with mayonnaise, sugar, and calories.
- Forgo the French fries and have baked, boiled, or roasted potatoes, or vegetables, but leave off the butter, cheese, and creams.
- Choose grilled, broiled, or baked meats and entrées.
- Drink water with your meal. Having water instead of soda, coffee, wine, or other alcoholic beverage helps you consume fewer calories, and less caffeine and sugar.
- Limit dessert. Try to satisfy your sweet tooth with low-fat desserts like fresh fruit, sorbet, sherbet, and nonfat frozen yogurt. If you do indulge in a high-calorie sweet, eat only a portion, or share it with the rest of the table.

＊ ●

HANDLING TRAVEL AND VACATIONS

- Eat at your usual times, without skipping meals. Drastically changing mealtimes can adversely affect your blood sugar control.
- When dining out, follow your meal plan as much as possible; always carry a snack in case there is a wait to be served.
- Carry with you a small bag of mixed nuts, hard-boiled eggs, or a few sticks of meat jerky; these foods help sustain blood sugar levels—especially on long car trips. If you have not eaten in a while, test your blood sugar prior to driving.
- Have on hand other portable between-meal snacks such as dried fruit, roasted soy nuts, or small packets of peanut butter.
- At airports, look for restaurants and snack bars that serve fruit, sushi, soup, or sandwiches.
- Order ahead. If your flight includes a meal, request a special diet such as a low-fat option or diet meal. Have water or juice rather than alcohol or soda (either can create blood sugar problems). Or bring your own food. A whole wheat bagel or crackers, a piece of fruit, a diabetic snack bar, and cut-up cheese and vegetables are healthy choices.
- At restaurants, make diet-friendly selections: grilled or roasted meats, chicken, or fish; steamed vegetables; salad with dressing on the side; and baked potato or steamed rice for carbohydrates rather than too much bread or other processed carbs.
- Make special requests for food that may not be on the menu. Many resorts provide dietary accommodations.
- Watch your serving sizes and always practice portion control.
- Keep snacks, juice, and/or glucose tablets close at hand to treat hypoglycemia.
- Limit your alcohol intake. If you opt to drink, eat food with your cocktail and choose drinks made with club soda or sugar-free soda.
- Never put your medicines in a checked suitcase. Always have direct access to insulin, oral medications, and diabetes supplies.
- Carry extra supplies, a written prescription, and the name of a doctor located at your destination.
- Carry a statement from your doctor verifying your diabetes and need for insulin and syringes. Always wear a medical alert tag.
- When crossing time zones, maintain your eating and insulin schedule according to your internal clock for a day before switching to the new time zone.
- For other helpful tips, log on to www.diabetictraveler.com.

✳

Recipes

Eggplant Dip

1 large eggplant, peeled and cut in quarters
2 cloves garlic, minced
1 scallion, chopped
½ cup chopped parsley
1 tablespoon lemon juice
½ teaspoon dill weed
10 black olives, pitted
Cucumber slices for dipping

✳ Place the eggplant pieces in a steamer basket and steam 10 to 15 minutes, until tender. When cool, press the liquid out of the eggplant. Place the cooked eggplant and all remaining ingredients except the olives into a blender and blend until smooth.

✳ Cut the olives into slivers and add to eggplant mixture. Chill before serving. Serve with cucumber slices for dipping.

MAKES 4 QUARTER-CUP SERVINGS

Nutrition information per serving: 27 calories, 1 gram protein, 4 grams carbohydrate, 1 gram fat, 2 grams fiber

Avocado and Tomato Salsa

1 ripe avocado, peeled, seeded, and diced
1 large tomato, diced (1½ cups)
½ cup diced yellow bell pepper
½ cup finely diced red onion
2 tablespoons fresh lime juice
1 jalapeño pepper, seeded and minced
1 clove garlic, minced
¼ cup (packed) fresh cilantro leaves, chopped

1 teaspoon freshly ground black pepper
Salt, to taste (optional)

✳ In a large bowl, combine avocado, tomato, bell pepper, onion, lime juice, jalapeño, garlic, cilantro, pepper, and salt (if used). Stir well.

✳ Serve promptly, accompanied by freshly chopped vegetables.

MAKES 6 SERVINGS

Nutrition information per serving: 72 calories, 2 grams protein, 10 grams carbohydrate, 4 grams fat, 3 grams fiber

BREAKFAST FOODS AND SMOOTHIES

Apple Smoothie

¼ cup applesauce
1 teaspoon ground cinnamon
1 banana
8 ounces unsweetened apple juice

✳ Place all ingredients in a blender and puree until smooth. Serve cold over ice.

MAKES 2 SERVINGS

Nutrition information per serving: 137 calories, 1 gram protein, 35 grams carbohydrate, <1 gram fat, 3 grams fiber

Raspberry Smoothie

1 cup plain nonfat yogurt
½ cup frozen unsweetened raspberries
½ cup orange juice

✳ Place all ingredients in a blender and puree until smooth.

MAKES 1 SERVING

Nutrition information per serving: 275 calories, 16 grams protein, 51 grams carbohydrate, 1 gram fat, 6 grams fiber

Strawberry-Orange Smoothie

1 cup frozen unsweetened strawberries
1 orange, peeled and sectioned
1 cup nonfat yogurt

✳ Place all ingredients in a blender and puree until smooth. Serve cold over ice.

MAKES 1 SERVING

Nutrition information per serving: 242 calories, 15 grams protein, 46 grams carbohydrate, 1 gram fat, 6 grams fiber

Tofu Colada

½ cup silken tofu
½ banana, frozen
½ teaspoon coconut extract
½ cup fresh pineapple chunks
½ cup skim milk
1 tablespoon honey

✳ Place all ingredients in a blender and puree until smooth.

MAKES 1 SERVING

Nutrition information per serving: 266 calories, 9 grams protein, 50 grams carbohydrate, 4 grams fat, 3 grams fiber

Oatmeal with Fruit

1½ cups unsweetened fruit juice
⅔ cup regular oatmeal
Pinch of salt
Pinch of ground cinnamon
⅓ cup minced dried peaches
1 tablespoon toasted wheat germ
1 cup low-fat milk

✳ In a small saucepan, combine juice, oatmeal, salt, and cinnamon. Heat to boiling. Reduce heat and simmer, uncovered, about 1 minute, until liquid is absorbed.

✳ Stir in peaches, cover pan, and let stand several minutes. Spoon into bowls, top with wheat germ, and serve hot with low-fat milk.

MAKES 2 SERVINGS

Nutrition information per serving: 432 calories, 18 grams protein, 850 grams carbohydrate, 5 grams fat, 7 grams fiber

Broiled Grapefruit

1 large grapefruit
Pinch of ground nutmeg
2 teaspoons dark brown sugar
2 teaspoons toasted wheat germ

✳ Heat broiler. Halve grapefruit and separate sections with a grapefruit knife. Sprinkle with nutmeg and brown sugar.

✳ Broil grapefruit 2 to 4 inches from heat for 3 to 4 minutes, until edges are browned a bit, sugar is melted, and grapefruit is heated through.

✳ Sprinkle with wheat germ and serve immediately.

MAKES 2 SERVINGS

Nutrition information per serving: 55 calories, 1 gram protein, 14 grams carbohydrate, 0 grams fat, 2 grams fiber

Oat Bran Bread French Toast

1 large egg
1 tablespoon skim milk
¼ teaspoon vanilla extract
Pinch of ground allspice
1 tablespoon canola oil
1 slice oat bran bread
No-sugar jam or no-sugar maple syrup for serving

✳ In a bowl, beat egg and milk with a fork. Add vanilla and allspice and beat until blended.

✳ Heat oil in a large nonstick skillet over medium heat. Dip bread in egg mixture and add to skillet. Cook about 3 to 4 minutes on each side, until browned on both sides, turning once. Serve hot with no-sugar jam or no-sugar maple syrup.

MAKES 1 SERVING

Nutrition information per serving: 280 calories, 10 grams protein, 14 grams carbohydrate, 21 grams fat, 1 gram fiber

Oat Bran Muffins

1 cup oat bran
1 cup all-purpose flour
1 tablespoon baking powder
1 tablespoon sugar
2 teaspoons grated lemon peel
½ teaspoon cream of tartar
½ teaspoon salt
⅓ cup canola oil
½ cup plain nonfat yogurt

✳ Heat oven to 425 degrees. Grind oat bran in a food processor about 2 minutes, until fine. Add flour, baking powder, sugar, lemon peel, cream of tartar, and salt. Process until completely mixed.

✳ Place flour mixture in a mixing bowl and stir in oil with a fork until it resembles coarse granules. Stir in yogurt until dough holds together. Turn out onto a lightly floured surface and gently knead the dough about 1 minute, until soft, smooth, and no longer sticky.

✳ Pat dough into an 8-inch square about ½ inch thick. Cut dough into 16 squares. Place them touching each other in two ungreased 8- or 9-inch cake pans. Bake for about 15 minutes, until browned and puffy.

MAKES 16 MUFFINS

Nutrition information per serving: 97 calories, 3 grams protein, 11 grams carbohydrate, 6 grams fat, 1 gram fiber

Black Bean Soup

2 tablespoons olive oil

2 medium onions, thinly sliced

2 cloves garlic, minced

2 16-ounce cans black beans, drained and rinsed

4 cups sodium-free chicken broth

1½ teaspoons ground cumin

½ teaspoon salt, or to taste

½ teaspoon dried oregano

½ teaspoon chili powder

Pinch of red pepper flakes

8 cherry tomatoes, seeded and cut into thin strips

2 scallions, minced

½ teaspoon grated lime peel, to taste

2 tablespoons minced fresh cilantro, plus 1 teaspoon for garnish

✳ Heat olive oil in a medium saucepan over medium heat. Add onions and cook about 5 minutes, until softened, stirring occasionally. Add garlic and cook about 3 minutes, stirring occasionally. Add beans, broth, cumin, salt, oregano, chili powder, and red pepper flakes. Heat to simmering; cook 10 minutes.

✳ Meanwhile, mix together cherry tomatoes, scallions, lime peel, and cilantro in a small bowl.

✳ Puree one cup of the soup mixture in a blender or food processor until smooth. Return to saucepan and stir to blend.

✳ Ladle soup into four bowls. Garnish each bowl with tomato mixture and sprinkle with cilantro. Serve hot.

MAKES 4 SERVINGS

Nutrition information per serving: 328 calories, 19 grams protein, 64 grams carbohydrate, 1 gram fat, 19 grams fiber

Creamy Broccoli Soup

2 cups canned low-sodium chicken broth
1 cup low-fat milk
1 tablespoon canola oil
1 cup chopped onion
2 cloves garlic, chopped
2 tablespoons unbleached all-purpose flour
6 cups chopped broccoli florets, cooked from frozen or fresh
1 cup (packed) Italian (flat-leaf) parsley leaves
1 tablespoon fresh thyme leaves
Salt and freshly ground black pepper, to taste

✳ In a small saucepan, heat chicken broth and milk until almost simmering. Meanwhile, in a large saucepan, heat oil over medium heat. Add onion and garlic and cook until translucent. Add flour and cook, stirring, 1 minute. Add hot broth mixture and simmer about 5 minutes, until mixture thickens, stirring constantly with whisk. Remove from heat and cool slightly.

✳ Carefully transfer mixture to a food processor, 2 to 3 cups at a time. Add broccoli, parsley, and thyme. Puree until smooth, in batches as necessary.

✳ Return soup to pan and reheat just to boiling. Season with salt and pepper to taste.

MAKES 4 SERVINGS

Nutrition information per serving: 182 calories, 8 grams protein, 29 grams carbohydrate, 5 grams fat, 8 grams fiber

Butternut Squash and Orange Soup

1 butternut squash (2 pounds), peeled and cut in 1-inch chunks (3½ cups)
1½ cups canned low-sodium chicken broth
½ teaspoon ground coriander
½ teaspoon cayenne
2 tablespoons orange juice, fresh or from concentrate
2 tablespoons (packed) Italian (flat-leaf) parsley leaves or cilantro
1 clove garlic, minced
1 teaspoon grated orange zest
½ teaspoon freshly ground black pepper

✳ In a medium saucepan, combine squash, broth, coriander, and cayenne. Bring to a boil, then reduce heat to low and simmer 10 to 15 minutes, until tender.

✳ Transfer mixture to a food processor. Add juice and process until smooth. Return to saucepan.

✳ Just before serving, chop together parsley or cilantro, garlic, orange zest, and pepper. Heat soup until almost boiling. Pour into serving bowls and sprinkle with zest mixture.

MAKES 4 SERVINGS

Nutrition information per serving: 95 calories, 4 grams protein, 20 grams carbohydrate, <1 gram fat, 6 grams fiber

VEGETABLE MAIN DISHES

Two-Minute Burritos

1 15-ounce can black beans	4 low-carb wheat tortillas
1 4-ounce can green chilies	2 to 4 tablespoons salsa

✳ In a saucepan, heat black beans and chilies (do not drain cans prior to heating). Remove from heat and drain juices.

✳ Spoon mixture into tortillas and top each one with 1 to 2 tablespoons salsa.

MAKES 2 SERVINGS

Nutrition information per serving: 445 calories, 21 grams protein, 78 grams carbohydrate, 6 grams fat, 18 grams fiber

Curried Garbanzo Beans

2 tablespoons canola oil

6 scallions, minced

1 teaspoon minced, peeled fresh ginger

1 clove garlic, minced

½ teaspoon curry powder

¼ teaspoon crushed red pepper flakes

1 16-ounce can garbanzo beans, rinsed and drained
1 4-ounce can minced roasted green chilies
¼ cup low-fat milk
½ teaspoon grated lime peel
1 tablespoon minced fresh cilantro

✳ Heat oil in a medium skillet over medium heat. Add scallions, ginger, garlic, and spices. Cook for 1 to 2 minutes, until very fragrant, stirring constantly.

✳ Add garbanzos and chilies and cook 3 minutes to heat through. Add milk and lime peel and cook for 2 to 3 minutes, stirring constantly. Sprinkle with cilantro and serve hot.

MAKES 4 SERVINGS

Nutrition information per serving: 218 calories, 6 grams protein, 30 grams carbohydrate, 9 grams fat, 6 grams fiber

Bell Pepper Lasagna

8 ounces whole wheat lasagna noodles (9 sheets)
1 tablespoon olive oil
2 medium onions, thinly sliced
4 red bell peppers, seeded and cut into ½-inch strips
4 green bell peppers, seeded and cut into ½-inch strips
Salt, to taste (optional)
Freshly ground black pepper, to taste
1 cup part-skim ricotta cheese
1 cup low-fat cottage cheese
2 large eggs, lightly beaten
½ teaspoon freshly ground black pepper
¼ cup (packed) fresh basil leaves, chopped
2 tablespoons nonfat Parmesan cheese
2½ cups no-sugar-added tomato sauce
1 cup shredded part-skim or nonfat mozzarella cheese

✳ Heat oven to 400 degrees.

✳ Cook lasagna noodles in plenty of water, until just tender. Drain and place them in cold water until needed.

✳ While pasta is cooking, heat oil in a large nonstick skillet over medium heat. Add onions and cook, stirring, until soft. Add bell peppers and cook about 15 minutes, until tender. Cover and continue cooking 10 minutes. Season with salt (if used) and pepper to taste.

✳ In a medium bowl, combine ricotta, cottage cheese, eggs, black pepper, basil, and Parmesan cheese.

✳ In a 12x9-inch lasagna pan or baking dish, spread ½ cup tomato sauce, then layer 3 noodles, ½ cup sauce, half ricotta mixture, half vegetable mixture, and ¼ cup mozzarella, repeat, ending with layer of 3 noodles. Spread top noodles with remaining 1 cup sauce and sprinkle with remaining cheese.

✳ Bake about 60 minutes, until cheese is melted and sauce is bubbly. Let lasagna stand for 10 minutes before cutting.

MAKES 8 SERVINGS

Nutrition information per serving: 250 calories, 15 grams protein, 30 grams carbohydrate, 8 grams fat, 3 grams fiber

Potato Kale Frittata

1 tablespoon olive oil
2 cups thinly sliced onion
3 cups chopped kale (12 ounces)
3 cloves garlic, minced
1 cup diced cooked potato
1 medium tomato, diced (1 cup)
1½ cups fat-free egg substitute
1 cup grated reduced-fat cheddar cheese (3 ounces)
½ cup tomato paste
½ teaspoon freshly ground black pepper, or to taste
Salt, to taste (optional)

✳ Heat broiler.

✳ Heat oil in a 10-inch, nonstick ovenproof skillet over medium-low heat. Add onion and cook, stirring, 7 to 8 minutes, until translucent. Add kale and garlic and cook until kale is wilted. Tilt pan to cover sides. Add potato and tomato, and toss gently.

* In a small bowl, stir egg substitute, cheese, tomato paste, pepper, and salt (if used) until well combined.

* Add egg mixture to hot skillet and smooth with a spatula. Continue cooking 5 to 6 minutes, until egg is almost set, lifting sides of frittata to allow raw egg to run underneath.

* Place skillet under broiler 4 to 5 minutes, to finish cooking. Slide frittata out onto plate, cut into wedges, and serve.

MAKES 4 SERVINGS

Nutrition information per serving: 268 calories, 15 grams protein, 38 grams carbohydrate, 6 grams fat, 4 grams fiber

MEAT, FISH, AND POULTRY MAIN DISHES

Shepherd's Pie with Sweet Potato Topping

2 baking potatoes, scrubbed

2 sweet potatoes, scrubbed

1 tablespoon canola oil

1 cup chopped onion

1 pound extra-lean ground beef

1½ cups canned reduced-sodium beef broth

8 canned tomatoes

1 tablespoon chopped fresh rosemary leaves

1 teaspoon chopped fresh thyme leaves

2 cups (packed) chopped fresh spinach (6 ounces)

* Heat oven to 400 degrees.

* Bake baking and sweet potatoes 45 to 60 minutes, until soft. Remove potatoes from oven. Reduce oven temperature to 375 degrees. When potatoes are cool enough to handle, peel. In a large bowl, combine potatoes and mash with a potato masher. Set aside.

* Heat oil in a large nonstick skillet over medium heat. Add onion and cook 5 to 6 minutes, stirring until it begins to brown. Reduce heat to medium. Add beef and continue cooking, stirring until beef is no longer pink. Add broth, tomatoes, rosemary, and thyme. Simmer 10 minutes.

✳ Add spinach and cook, stirring, until spinach is just wilted. Remove from heat.

✳ Transfer mixture to a 6-cup baking dish and spoon mashed potatoes over the top of the mixture, covering completely. Bake about 45 minutes, until top is golden.

MAKES 4 SERVINGS

Nutrition information per serving: 433 calories, 28 grams protein, 41 grams carbohydrate, 17 grams fat, 6 grams fiber

Beefsteak with Tomato-Orange Salsa

2 medium tomatoes, diced (2 cups)
1 cup thinly sliced red onion
1 cup orange sections
1 tablespoon olive oil
1 teaspoon chopped fresh thyme leaves
¼ teaspoon cayenne
Salt, to taste (optional)
4 beefsteaks, such as London broil (5 ounces each)

✳ In a medium bowl, combine tomatoes, onion, orange sections, olive oil, thyme, cayenne, and salt (if used). Cover and set aside for 30 minutes.

✳ Broil steaks 4 inches from heat for 10 to 20 minutes each side, to desired doneness. Serve topped with salsa.

MAKES 4 SERVINGS

Nutrition information per serving: 228 calories, 26 grams protein, 11 grams carbohydrate, 8 grams fat, 3 grams fiber

Baked Tuna Steaks with Peppers and Mushrooms

1 cup thinly sliced red onion
4 bell peppers (a mixture of green, red, and yellow), sliced in thin strips
4 cloves garlic, minced
1 cup shiitake mushrooms, thinly sliced
4 tuna steaks (5 ounces each)

½ cup dry white wine or vegetable broth
2 tablespoons fresh lemon juice
½ teaspoon freshly ground black pepper

✳ Heat oven to 450 degrees. Combine onion, peppers, garlic, and mushrooms in a baking dish large enough for tuna steaks to fit in a single layer. Place tuna steaks on top.

✳ Mix wine, lemon juice, and pepper, and pour over fish. Cover tightly with foil and make a few small holes in the foil. Bake about 20 minutes, until fish is cooked through.

MAKES 4 SERVINGS

Nutrition information per serving: 235 calories, 27 grams protein, 23 grams carbohydrate, 2 grams fat, 4 grams fiber

Oven "Fried" Fish

4 cups whole wheat bread crumbs
4 egg whites
½ cup skim milk
1 pound ocean perch fillets or other white fish
Vegetable cooking spray

✳ Process bread crumbs in a blender until fine. Set aside.

✳ In a small bowl, beat egg whites and skim milk until well blended. Dip fillets into egg mixture, then roll in bread crumbs, coating both sides.

✳ Spread fillets on a cookie sheet that has been sprayed several times with vegetable cooking spray. Lightly coat fillets with spray. Bake at 400 degrees for 20 minutes.

MAKES 4 SERVINGS

Nutrition information per serving: 230 calories, 26 grams protein, 26 grams carbohydrate, 2 grams fat, 1 gram fiber

Fish in Spicy Tomato Sauce

1 tablespoon olive oil
1 cup chopped onion
2 cloves garlic, minced
¾ cup dry white wine
1 28-ounce can whole plum tomatoes in juice, coarsely chopped
1 cup water
1 teaspoon grated orange zest
¼ to ½ teaspoon hot pepper flakes
1 sprig fresh rosemary
4 cod fillets (5 ounces each)

✳ Heat oil over medium-high heat in a large nonstick skillet. Add onion and cook, stirring, 4 to 5 minutes, until tender. Add garlic and cook 1 minute. Add wine and continue cooking until evaporated.

✳ Add tomatoes and juice, water, orange zest, pepper flakes, and whole rosemary sprig. Simmer 15 minutes, until thickened.

✳ Nestle fish fillets in tomato sauce. Partially cover and cook until fish is just cooked through, 4 to 8 minutes, depending on thickness. Serve fillets topped with sauce, first removing rosemary sprig.

MAKES 4 SERVINGS

Nutrition information per serving: 224 calories, 22 grams protein, 21 grams carbohydrate, 4 grams fat, 3 grams fiber

Chicken Parmigiana

2 cups whole wheat bread crumbs
¾ cup grated fat-free Parmesan cheese
3 egg whites
½ cup skim milk
1 pound boneless, skinless chicken breasts
Vegetable cooking spray

✳ Process bread crumbs in a blender until fine and stir in Parmesan cheese. Set aside.

✳ In a small bowl, beat egg whites and skim milk until well blended. Dip chicken into egg mixture, then roll in bread crumb mixture, coating both sides.

✳ Spread chicken on a cookie sheet that has been sprayed several times with vegetable cooking spray. Lightly coat chicken with spray. Bake at 400 degrees for 25 minutes.

MAKES 4 SERVINGS

Nutrition information per serving: 275 calories, 34 grams protein, 20 grams carbohydrate, 6 grams fat, <1 gram fiber

MAIN DISH SALADS

Salmon and Vegetable Salad

4 red potatoes, peeled and quartered

2 cups string beans, cut into 1-inch lengths

½ cup plain nonfat yogurt

2 shallots, minced

2 tablespoons minced fresh dill

1 tablespoon Dijon mustard

¼ teaspoon salt

¼ teaspoon freshly ground black pepper

2 cups grated zucchini

1 cup canned small white beans, rinsed and drained

4 carrots, grated

1 cup finely shredded red cabbage

1 7½-ounce can water-packed salmon, drained

10 radishes, sliced

4 tablespoons olive oil

2 tablespoons minced fresh parsley

✳ Cook potatoes in boiling water about 20 to 25 minutes, until done. Blanch string beans by adding them to the potato water about 4 minutes before draining potatoes.

✳ Meanwhile, make yogurt dressing: Whisk yogurt, shallots, dill, Dijon mustard, salt, and black pepper.

✳ Add remaining ingredients to potatoes and string beans. Toss well to combine. Stir in yogurt mixture and blend. Serve at room temperature or chilled.

MAKES 4 SERVINGS

Nutrition information per serving: 422 calories, 12 grams protein, 65 grams carbohydrate, 14 grams fat, 14 grams fiber

Tuna Niçoise Salad

1 3-ounce can tuna
½ cup cooked string beans (cold)
1 small boiled potato, sliced
Lettuce
2 tablespoons low-fat Italian dressing

✳ Arrange tuna, beans, and potato on a bed of lettuce. Drizzle with dressing.

MAKES 1 SERVING

Nutrition information per serving: 300 calories, 27 grams protein, 44 grams carbohydrate, 2 grams fat, 7 grams fiber

Shrimp and Rice Salad

16 ounces medium shrimp, peeled, deveined, and cooked
3 cups cooked brown rice
3 red bell peppers, roasted and diced (from a jar)
⅓ cup sliced red onion
¼ cup (packed) Italian (flat-leaf) parsley, chopped
2 tablespoons chopped fresh thyme leaves
2 tablespoons fresh lemon juice
1 tablespoon olive oil
1 tablespoon white vinegar
½ teaspoon Dijon mustard
Freshly ground black pepper, to taste
Bibb lettuce leaves

✳ In a large bowl, combine shrimp, rice, peppers, onion, and parsley. Set aside.

✳ In a small bowl, combine thyme, lemon juice, oil, vinegar, mustard, and pepper. Whisk vigorously until well blended. Toss with rice mixture. Serve on lettuce leaves.

MAKES 4 SERVINGS

Nutrition information per serving: 270 calories, 22 grams protein, 42 grams carbohydrate, 1 gram fat, 1 gram fiber

Chicken Wild Rice Salad with Mango

5 cups canned low-sodium chicken broth
1 cup wild rice, rinsed and drained
2 cups shredded, cooked chicken breast
2 large ripe mangoes, peeled and diced (2 cups)
1 medium tomato, sliced
1 red bell pepper, seeded and diced
1 cup diced cucumber
¼ cup thinly sliced scallions
2 tablespoons chopped walnuts
⅓ cup orange juice, fresh or from concentrate
2 tablespoons olive oil
1 teaspoon white vinegar
1½ teaspoons grated peeled fresh ginger
½ teaspoon freshly ground black pepper
Salt, to taste (optional)

✳ In a medium saucepan, bring broth to boiling. Stir in wild rice, reduce heat to low, and simmer, uncovered, about 45 minutes, until tender. Drain well and cool to room temperature.

✳ In a large bowl, combine rice, chicken, mangoes, tomato, red pepper, cucumber, scallions, and walnuts.

✳ In a separate bowl, combine orange juice, oil, vinegar, ginger, pepper, and salt (if used). Toss with the mango mixture.

MAKES 4 SERVINGS

Nutrition information per serving: 323 calories, 29 grams protein, 30 grams carbohydrate, 11 grams fat, 4 grams fiber

Braised Red Cabbage with Apple

1 tablespoon canola oil
1 medium onion, minced
½ small head red cabbage, shredded
1 Golden Delicious apple, pared, cored, and finely diced
½ cup fat-free chicken broth
¼ cup plus 5 tablespoons dry white wine
1 teaspoon Dijon mustard
½ teaspoon sugar
¼ teaspoon grated lime peel
¼ teaspoon freshly ground pepper
¼ teaspoon salt

✳ Heat oil in a medium nonstick skillet over medium heat. Add onion and sauté about 4 minutes, until softened, stirring occasionally.

✳ Add remaining ingredients and cook about 15 minutes, until cabbage is softened and most of the cooking liquid is absorbed, stirring occasionally. Serve hot.

MAKES 2 SERVINGS

Nutrition information per serving: 205 calories, 4 grams protein, 23 grams carbohydrate, 7 grams fat, 4 grams fiber

Scallion Corn Bread

1 cup all-purpose flour
¾ cup cornmeal
¼ cup oat bran
1 teaspoon salt
1 teaspoon baking powder
½ teaspoon baking soda
1 cup plain nonfat yogurt
2 large eggs, or equivalent egg substitute
¼ cup canola oil
2 scallions, minced

✳ Heat oven to 350 degrees. In a medium bowl, mix flour, cornmeal, oat bran, salt, baking powder, and baking soda.

✳ In another medium bowl, whisk together remaining ingredients until thoroughly blended. Add cornmeal mixture and mix well. Pour batter into a greased 10-inch cast-iron skillet.

✳ Bake about 35 minutes, until top is browned and a wooden pick inserted in center comes out clean. Cool on a wire rack. Serve warm, if desired.

MAKES 10 SERVINGS

Nutrition information per serving: 177 calories, 6 grams protein, 23 grams carbohydrate, 7 grams fat, 2 grams fiber

Baked Sweet Potato Fries

4 sweet potatoes, scrubbed
Vegetable cooking spray
1 tablespoon sesame seed
Salt, to taste (optional)

✳ Heat oven to 450 degrees.

✳ Cut unpeeled potatoes lengthwise into ⅓-inch slices. Cut into sticks. Spray potatoes with vegetable oil spray until well coated, then toss with sesame seed and salt (if used).

✳ Transfer potatoes to a cookie sheet coated with vegetable spray. Bake 15 minutes; turn and continue baking 15 to 20 minutes, until golden.

MAKES 4 SERVINGS

Nutrition information per serving: 144 calories, 3 grams protein, 30 grams carbohydrate, 2 grams fat, 5 grams fiber

Sautéed Broccoli and Garlic

4 tablespoons olive oil
4 cloves garlic, finely slivered
4 cups broccoli florets, thawed from frozen
Salt, to taste (optional)
Freshly ground black pepper, to taste

✳ Heat oil in a large nonstick skillet over medium heat. Add garlic and cook for 30 seconds, stirring constantly.

✳ Add broccoli and continue cooking until garlic is golden.

✳ Toss with salt (if used) and pepper. Remove from heat.

MAKES 4 SERVINGS

Nutrition information per serving: 175 calories, 6 grams protein, 10 grams carbohydrate, 14 grams fat, 6 grams fiber

Strawberries in Balsamic Vinegar

4 cups strawberries
¼ cup honey
2 tablespoons balsamic vinegar

✳ Hull strawberries and cut into halves.

✳ In a medium bowl, combine berries and honey and let stand 30 minutes before serving. Sprinkle with vinegar and gently toss to blend. Serve immediately.

MAKES 4 SERVINGS

Nutrition information per serving: 117 calories, 1 gram protein, 30 grams carbohydrate, <1 gram fat, 3 grams fiber

Rice Pudding

1 cup skim milk
1 large egg, lightly beaten, or equivalent egg substitute
4 dried peaches, diced
1 tablespoon dried currants
1 tablespoon honey
Pinch of ground cinnamon
1 cup cooked brown rice (½ cup uncooked)

✳ In a small saucepan, stir all ingredients, except rice, until well blended.

✳ Stir in cooked rice and cook mixture over medium heat 7 to 10 minutes, until thickened, stirring frequently. Serve warm.

MAKES 2 SERVINGS

Nutrition information per serving: 333 calories, 12 grams protein, 60 grams carbohydrate, 5 grams fat, 4 grams fiber

Sweet Potato Custard

4 medium sweet potatoes
2 tablespoons light brown sugar
¼ cup orange juice, fresh or from concentrate
4 teaspoons fresh lemon juice
1 cup plain yogurt

✳ Heat oven to 400 degrees.

✳ Bake potatoes about 45 minutes, until soft. Cool completely.

✳ Remove potato pulp from skin and place in a medium bowl. Add sugar and juices. Beat with an electric mixer until sugar is dissolved and potatoes are light. Fold in yogurt.

✳ Transfer mixture to custard cups. Refrigerate 1 hour, until cold.

MAKES 4 SERVINGS

Nutrition information per serving: 150 calories, 6 grams protein, 40 grams carbohydrate, 4 grams fat, 5 grams fiber

The Promise of
Complementary Therapy

IN A SOCIETY LIKE OURS WHERE FOOD
and nutrients are so plentiful, does anyone really need to take vitamins, minerals, or herbs? If you have prediabetes or diabetes, should you take them? If so, which ones and how much? When it comes to dietary supplements and other forms of complementary and alternative medicine (CAM), the answers are often unclear and confusing, especially with so many ads promising such dramatic results.

More than sixty-five years ago, the U.S. government established recommended daily allowances (RDAs) for most vitamins and minerals. The RDA specifies the daily amount of nutrients we need to maintain health, based on age and gender. It also represents the amount required to prevent certain nutritional deficiency diseases, such as scurvy and rickets. As our knowledge of nutrition expanded, so did the method of rating the amounts of nutrients we need for good health. We now use what is termed the Dietary Reference Intakes (DRIs). This includes the RDA, as well as two other rating systems:

a set of values called tolerable upper intake levels, which sets ceilings to help us avoid taking too much of a nutrient; and adequate intakes, or AI, an estimate of average intake that is healthy and won't harm health. Most dietitians and medical experts describe nutrient recommendations in terms of DRIs.

Even so, there are those who claim that taking megadoses—amounts in excess of DRIs—will cure diseases. Most of these claims are made on the basis of flimsy scientific data, and unfortunately many people are willing to embrace worthless or unproven treatments in the hope that they may be cured.

I feel like I am in a unique position to help you sift through the often conflicting data on supplements and diabetes based on my experience in this field and interest in various botanical and nutritional supplements. I can also tell you that rigorous scientific research on CAM, including supplements, is taking place at major academic and medical institutions throughout the United States. For example, the National Institutes of Health (NIH) has established and funded several research centers devoted exclusively to the study and evaluation of natural products, not only for their effects on obesity and carbohydrate metabolism, but also for other health-related conditions. Some of the agents being tested for diabetes have been used traditionally by many cultures for centuries, others are rather new on the scene. Some of the nutrients under evaluation are familiar, like chromium, vitamin C, and vitamin E. Others, such as Russian tarragon, are unfamiliar. The point is, scientists are taking these agents seriously and beginning to understand what works and what doesn't. This information ultimately helps you make better, more informed health decisions.

From my experience, research, and review of the available published studies, it appears that there are specific agents showing promise as "adjunctive," or "*added in*" therapy if you have prediabetes or diabetes. These are supplements that you may want to try, *but only in consultation with your physician.* Generally, these substances and supplements have been tested more rigorously through controlled clinical trials and double-blind studies, and found to be helpful for the specific conditions for which their use is proposed. In other words, they may be worth adding to your daily regimen. Approaches that include a multiple vitamin/mineral supplement, fish oils, or perhaps chromium may fall into this category. In addition, there is supplemental magnesium, which is strictly indicated only in the case of a diagnosed magnesium deficiency. A prescription form of the B-vitamin niacin, used to treat lipid disorders, is available too, but clearly is not appropriate for everyone and should be considered only after consultation with your physician.

There are many other substances, including numerous botanicals (herbs) that are promoted as remedies for diabetes, but have limited scientific data to support their claims. I want you to be aware of these too, so that you don't spend your money needlessly or take something that could harm your health. Because of the lack of adequate research data showing effectiveness and safety, I have placed these in a category called "can't yet be recommended." Herbs may be "natural," but just because they are labeled as such, don't be fooled by this claim. In fact, many products promoted as being "natural" may have potentially harmful side effects. Some supplements, for example, may adversely affect your blood sugar control or cause drug interactions. I hope that the information in this chapter will help you sort through the confusion regarding supplements. Additionally, at the end of the chapter, I'll provide information for several other forms of complementary therapy referred to as "mind-body medicine."

What follows, then, is a look at supplements that may help you when used sensibly, and supplements that are not yet considered helpful in treating diabetes. Some important words of advice: never substitute a vitamin, mineral, or any form of supplement for a healthy lifestyle or for your prescription diabetes medication. And always tell your doctor if you are taking nutritional supplements.

Promising? Worth Trying Now?

Multiple Vitamin/Mineral/Antioxidant Supplements

In the human body, vitamins and minerals play a vital role in helping regulate the chemical reactions that govern cells and convert food into energy and living tissue. Certain nutrients like vitamin C and some minerals act as antioxidants, protecting your cells against highly reactive molecules, called free radicals, that destroy tissue. Some vitamins are manufactured within the body. Vitamin D, for example, is made in the skin when it is exposed to sunlight, and three other vitamins (K, biotin, and pantothenic acid) are made inside the human gut by resident bacteria. But most vitamins must be obtained through the foods you eat, particularly by consuming fruits and vegetables on a daily basis—a good health habit with merits across the board. The problem is, only a mere 9 percent of adults manage to consume the recommended daily amount of fruits and vegetables, according to the National Center for Health Statistics. Taking vitamins and minerals in pill form helps fill in the gaps, and most doctors today endorse this practice.

MULTIPLE VITAMIN/MINERAL/ANTIOXIDANT SUPPLEMENTS AND DIABETES

The American Diabetes Association states that individuals with diabetes should be aware of the importance of acquiring daily vitamin and mineral requirements from natural food sources and a balanced diet. However, depending on how balanced your diet may be, if you have diabetes, supplementing with a daily multiple vitamin tablet may be a good idea. For example, a randomized, double-blind, placebo-controlled trial of 130 people with diabetes showed that those who took a multivitamin and mineral supplement reported fewer infectious illnesses and fewer days lost from work than did those in the placebo group. This study was published in the *Annals of Internal Medicine* in 2003. In this regard, the daily multiple vitamin tablet is not providing megadoses of vitamins, but is simply designed to make sure your daily intake is on par with what your body requires on a daily basis.

DOSAGE: HOW MUCH?

I feel that it is important to use a daily multiple vitamin tablet to support a nutritious, well-rounded diet, like the ones outlined for you in chapters 4 and 5.

Multiple vitamin/mineral supplements are typically formulated in a harmonious balance designed to ensure absorption and effectiveness. You'll want to select a product containing 100 percent of the daily requirement for vitamins and minerals, and take it only once a day. Also, choose a multiple vitamin formulation that carries the USP (United States Pharmacopeia) certification on the label. These factors assure a certain degree of quality control. Your doctor, pharmacist, or diabetes educator can help you select a good product.

Niacin

Niacin is a member of the B-complex family of vitamins, which are involved in a wide variety of metabolic functions, including energy production within cells, cholesterol and carbohydrate metabolism, and the production of hormones. The best food sources of niacin are meats, poultry, fish, and wheat germ.

NIACIN AND DIABETES

For many years now, high doses of niacin have been promoted to help reduce cholesterol and triglycerides. This form of therapy also helps raise beneficial HDL ("good" cholesterol), making it attractive to people with type 2 diabetes, who are at a higher risk for heart disease. Technically, niacin is a vitamin, but when used in the high doses required to regulate blood lipids, it is considered a drug. Higher-dose niacin is available as a prescription drug called Niaspan.

Niaspan can be beneficial when added to statin therapy (for controlling cholesterol) if you have diabetes. In one study, 148 patients were randomized to 1,000 or 1,500 milligrams a day of niacin, or a placebo. About half the participants continued their prescribed cholesterol-lowering statin drugs during the study, and 81 percent kept taking their oral medications for diabetes. By the end of the sixteen-week experimental period, HDL ("good" cholesterol) increased and triglycerides fell in those taking the high-dose niacin. *However, do not begin niacin until talking with your physician.* The reasons are that high-dose niacin when combined with other cholesterol-lowering drugs may increase the symptoms such as muscle weakness, pain, or tenderness and these may be the signs of a serious but rare side effect. In addition, there needs to be close follow-up because higher-dose niacin may indeed worsen your blood sugar. *So, this is not a supplement that you should take without first discussing it with your medical provider.*

DOSAGE: HOW MUCH?

Higher-dose niacin is generally given by prescription. The usual starting dose is one 500-milligram tablet daily. Every four weeks, your doctor may increase your dosage by 500 milligrams, up to a maximum dosage of 2,000 milligrams taken once a day, depending on your response to the drug. Your doctor should monitor your treatment carefully, since combination therapy may result in more side effects.

PRECAUTIONS

You should not self-medicate by taking over-the-counter niacin. Talk to your doctor about whether you are even a candidate for niacin.

One of the other problems with niacin is the flushing. Flushing is caused by a sudden expansion of the small blood vessels at the surface of the skin, termed vasodilation. It may seem alarming if you're not expecting it. For most people, it is mild to moderate, and tends to lessen over time. You can further minimize flushing by taking aspirin or ibuprofen (with your doctor's approval), or taking niacin at bedtime. Niaspan may help minimize flushing, the major side effect of high-dose niacin. Also, if you are prescribed Niaspan, you'll have to keep a sharp eye on your blood sugar, since this drug may increase it. So, despite the benefit this therapy can provide you, there are also risks if you have diabetes.

Chromium

One of the most common elements in the earth's crust and seawater, chromium exists in our environment in three principal forms: metallic, trivalent, and hexavalent chromium. Trivalent chromium, found in most foods and dietary supplements, is an essential nutrient. Meat and whole-grain products, as well as brewer's yeast and certain spices, are relatively good sources. Chromium is also present in many multivitamin/mineral supplements, and it is marketed by itself in supplement form (capsules and tablets) as chromium picolinate, chromium chloride, and chromium nicotinate. Next to calcium, chromium is the most popular supplement sold in the United

States. An adequate intake of chromium is approximately 25 to 35 micrograms a day.

CHROMIUM AND DIABETES

Some researchers say chromium may enhance the action of insulin in the body. Because of this connection, chromium is being looked at as a possible adjunctive therapy in diabetes. The interest in chromium for enhancing glucose metabolism can be traced back to the 1950s, when it was suggested that brewer's yeast contained a glucose tolerance factor (GTF) that was an effective treatment for diabetes in experimental animals.

Further interest in giving chromium to patients with diabetes was kindled by the observation in the 1970s that it truly was an essential nutrient required for normal carbohydrate metabolism. Patients receiving total parenteral nutrition (TPN) in the hospital developed severe signs of diabetes, including hyperglycemia (high blood sugar). When subsequently given supplemental chromium, in a relatively short time, the signs and symptoms of diabetes improved. Other studies of the beneficial effects of chromium in patients receiving TPN have also been documented in the scientific literature. Chromium is now routinely added to TPN solutions. However, most people are not considered chromium deficient, so the role of supplemental chromium to improve glucose is still controversial.

Research into chromium and diabetes has been a research interest of mine, since the mineral is believed to help cells process insulin more effectively (insulin sensitivity). In an early study, my colleagues and I evaluated individuals who were considered at high risk for type 2 diabetes because of their family history and obesity. In this double-blind, randomized, placebo-controlled trial, the subjects took chromium picolinate (1,000 micrograms a day) or a placebo for eight months. The chromium-supplement group showed a significant increase in insulin sensitivity midway through the study, whereas the placebo group had no significant changes. In that study, we didn't find any effect of chromium picolinate on body weight, abdominal fat, or body mass index (BMI), a measure of weight relative to height and waist circumference. Improvement in insulin sensitivity without a change in body fat distribution suggested that chromium may affect insulin independently of changes in body weight.

In another study, we looked into the effect of chromium picolinate on insulin sensitivity, blood sugar control, and body composition in twenty-nine people with type 2 diabetes. They took an oral diabetes drug called Glucotrol (5 milligrams a day) and a placebo for three months. Next, they were randomized in a double-blind fashion to receive either the drug plus the placebo, or the drug plus chromium picolinate (1,000 micrograms a day) for six months. We measured their body composition, insulin sensitivity, and blood sugar control at the start of the study, at the end of the three-month single-blind placebo phase, and at the end of the study.

Here is what we observed: from the time we began the study, the people who took the drug and the placebo gained weight, body fat, and abdominal fat; those taking the drug and chromium picolinate had less weight gain. Also, those taking the drug and chromium picolinate had significant improvements in insulin sensitivity and free fatty acids, as opposed to Glucotrol plus the placebo. We concluded from this study that adding chromium picolinate to diabetes drug therapy (Glucotrol) optimized insulin activity and blood sugar control. Further, chromium picolinate supplements significantly helped prevent weight gain, including abdominal fat, compared with the placebo group.

Other studies such as those done by Dr. Richard Anderson have shown positive effects with chromium picolinate in patients with diabetes. In one of his studies, blood sugar control improved in people who took 200 or 1,000 micrograms a day.

However, other investigators have not confirmed these effects, suggesting that chromium may not be beneficial. Recently, a research study conducted in Europe by Dr. Nanne Kleefstra suggested that chromium supplementation had no effect in individuals with type 2 diabetes. The reasons for the discrepancy in the findings are clearly of interest, and it certainly may be that some patient variables, such as obesity and insulin resistance, may predict who will or will not respond. These types of studies are currently ongoing, and the answer will be critical to determine who will and will not respond to chromium supplementation.

DOSAGE: HOW MUCH?

If you are diabetic and trying to control blood sugar the addition of chromium to your regimen will need to be discussed with your provider. As stated, some studies have suggested it may help, where as others have not. Although studies have used as high as 1,000 micrograms a day, Dr. Anderson's studies suggested some benefit as low as 200 micrograms. As of now, 200 to 400 micrograms a day may be a reasonable dose and should not be used in place of any of your prescription meds, but only considered as "adjunctive" therapy, or added to your current diabetes meds, under the supervision of your medical provider.

PRECAUTIONS

There have been concerns regarding the long-term safety of chromium supplementation. These stemmed from the results of studies in which huge doses of chromium picolinate inflicted DNA damage in cells cultured in lab dishes. However, to date, there is no evidence that chromium does this in the body. Chromium picolinate has also been associated with a few serious adverse reactions, including kidney failure, but the relationship of chromium to these events is not clear. Reviews of the safety of chromium picolinate by the Institute of Medicine have concluded that the supplement appears safe. If you decide to use this supplement, and given the fact it may affect your blood sugar, inform your physician that you are taking it and have him or her monitor your condition carefully. Chromium supplements are not designed to replace medication prescribed for blood sugar control.

Magnesium

Magnesium is a mineral that has many important functions in the body, including in the heart, nerves, muscles, bones, handling glucose, and manufacturing proteins. It is found in green leafy vegetables, nuts, seeds, and some whole grains. Adequate dietary intakes for both men and women range from 300 to 400 milligrams a day. Various supplemental forms of magnesium are marketed as tablets, capsules, or liquids.

MAGNESIUM AND DIABETES

Evidence is showing up that suboptimal levels of magnesium are linked to a number of disorders, including insulin resistance, type 2 diabetes, high blood pressure, and cardiovascular disease. Some research suggests that if you get enough magnesium from your diet, your risk of developing type 2 diabetes goes down. So there seems to be a connection between magnesium levels in the body and diabetes.

Does this mean you need to supplement with magnesium?

Possibly—but only if you have type 2 diabetes *and* are magnesium depleted. That's the suggestion of a recent randomized double-blind, placebo-controlled study involving sixty-three patients with a magnesium deficiency who were being treated with a drug called glibenclamide, an agent that works to release increased amounts of insulin from the pancreas. The patients received either a magnesium supplement or a placebo each day for sixteen weeks. By the end of the study, the supplement takers reduced their fasting glucose levels and lowered their A1c, plus increased the amount of magnesium in their bodies. The results suggest that glucose control, if associated with a magnesium deficiency, may be improved with magnesium supplementation.

DOSAGE: HOW MUCH?

The American Diabetes Association says that there is no benefit to supplementing with magnesium if you are diabetic unless you're deficient in this mineral. You can have your magnesium levels checked through blood testing. If you are deficient, your doctor may prescribe a magnesium supplement. But, generally with a well-balanced diet, and particularly if you take a daily vitamin/mineral tablet, you will most likely NOT be magnesium deficient and the overwhelming majority of patients do quite well without taking any additional magnesium supplements.

PRECAUTIONS

Anyone who is diabetic and takes a magnesium supplement should do so only under the supervision of a doctor.

Omega-3 Fatty Acids

Omega-3 fatty acids (omega-3s, for short) are a group of polyunsaturated fatty acids that come from food sources, such as fish, fish oil, some vegetable oils (such as canola and soybean), walnuts, and certain dietary supplements. As supplements, omega-3s are marketed as capsules or oils, often as fish oil. Omega-3s are important in a number of bodily functions, including making our cell membranes more flexible, the relaxation and contraction of muscles, blood clotting, digestion, fertility, cell division, and growth. Unfortunately, humans are unable to make these fatty acids, and we must get them from food we eat. As stated above, cold-water fish, such as salmon, are rich in omega-3 fatty acids.

OMEGA-3S AND DIABETES

Omega-3s have been the focus of much attention in recent years because of research showing they may decrease the rate of heart disease, reduce inflammation, and lower triglyceride levels. Omega-3s have been of interest to diabetics, since having this disease increases the risk of heart disease and stroke. Since 2004, the Food and Drug Administration (FDA) has allowed food companies to make certain claims about the heart-healthy benefits of omega-3 fatty acids on their packages. The FDA concluded that while these particular fatty acids are not essential to the diet, they may be beneficial in reducing coronary heart disease. The agency determined there was enough scientific evidence to allow companies to make what are known as qualified health claims, which can be included on food labels based on a preponderance of research results and usually refer to a specific health benefit—in the case of omega-3s, that they may reduce the risk of coronary heart disease.

DOSAGE: HOW MUCH?

Talk to your doctor about whether you should supplement with omega-3s. The American Diabetes Association recommends two to three servings of fish per week in order to obtain adequate amounts of omega-3 fatty acids. The American Heart Association has published similar recommendations. So, clearly, eating fish two or three times a week is a good way to boost your intake of these fats.

PRECAUTIONS

Fish oil supplements, in particular, taken in high doses can possibly interact with and influence the action of certain medications, including blood thinners (like Coumadin) and drugs for high blood pressure. Potential side effects of fish oil supplements include a fishy aftertaste, belching, stomach disturbances, and nausea. So, once again, there is clearly benefit for omega-3 fatty acids particularly when consumed as part of a healthy diet with the recommended fish servings per week. Whether you need to supplement above this is, once again, something that will need to be done in consultation with your medical provider.

Can't Yet Be Recommended

The following supplements, including botanicals, have some preliminary research behind them, but there is not yet enough data to suggest taking them until more is known.

Vitamin C

Vitamin C is a major player in the formation of connective tissue such as collagen. It is also involved in boosting immunity, wound healing, and cholesterol reduction.

VITAMIN C AND DIABETES

Vitamin C has been in the nutritional spotlight for a long time, for everything from reducing infections to helping with heart disease. In heart disease, researchers have looked into the effect of vitamin C on a condition called endothelial dysfunction. Let me explain: there are special cells in the blood vessels called endothelial cells; they line the inner surface of all blood vessels, including your arteries and veins. These cells have many vital jobs in your body: they regulate normal blood clotting, enhance immunity, and control the comings and goings of electrolytes inside and outside cells. Events like smoking, high blood pressure, abnormal cholesterol, and diabetes interfere with their cellular duties. When endothelial cells can't perform their jobs, your arteries are unable to dilate normally and their production of favorable chemicals may be altered. These abnormalities may trigger atherosclerosis (the narrowing of the arteries that increases the risk of heart attacks). In people who are insulin resistant and who have prediabetes, endothelial function appears to be impaired. There are several small scale studies showing that large doses of vitamin C , or more prolonged treatment, for example, 500 milligrams of vitamin C taken daily for thirty days, may improve endothelial dysfunction associated with diabetes. More research, however, is needed to confirm a benefit.

PRECAUTIONS

There is no question that vitamin C is an important nutrient. You can easily get the recommended amounts—75 milligrams a day for women and 90 milligrams for men—from a diet that is rich in fruits and vegetables. The American Diabetes Association cautions people to avoid megadosing on any antioxidants, including vitamin C. I agree, so I would suggest not taking megadoses of this supplement until more is known about it. If you eat a healthy diet and take a multiple vitamin preparation, you should have adequate intake of vitamin C.

Vitamin E

Vitamin E is one of the fat-soluble vitamins, meaning that it is stored in the fatty tissues of the body. It is an antioxidant believed to protect cells from free-radical damage.

VITAMIN E AND DIABETES

In high doses (200 IU or above), vitamin E has been promoted as effective for forestalling certain complications of diabetes, such as heart disease, kidney problems, nerve disease, and eye disease. But does it actually confer these benefits?

Some research hints that:

- In people with type 2 diabetes, vitamin E may help reduce LDL ("bad" cholesterol), possibly preventing cardiovascular disease or at least keep it from progressing.
- Vitamin E may improve kidney function and endothelial function in people with type 1 diabetes.
- Vitamin E may be beneficial against small blood vessel disease that involves the retina and the kidneys, and therefore may provide a health hedge against these complications.
- Vitamin E may reduce glucose, LDL ("bad" cholesterol), total cholesterol, triglycerides, and A1c.

The above data is certainly good news, but more studies are needed. What's more, I do need to bring to your attention a fairly recent study that evaluated whether long-term supplementation with vitamin E could decrease the risk of cancer, cancer death, and major cardiovascular events. This large double-blind, placebo-controlled trial was called the Heart Outcomes

Prevention Evaluation, and it was published in *The Journal of the American Medical Association* in 2005. Essentially, it found that taking 400 IUs of vitamin E each day *did nothing* to prevent heart attacks or stroke. In patients with vascular disease or diabetes, long-term vitamin E supplementation did not prevent cancer either, and may even increase the risk for heart failure.

PRECAUTIONS

As a result of studies like the one mentioned above, be cautious about taking vitamin E supplements. Instead, obtain the recommended dietary intake of vitamin E (15 milligrams daily) from food sources such as avocados, nuts, and vegetable oils.

Also, supplemental vitamin E has an anticoagulant effect. It promotes factors in the blood that can increase bleeding and thus should not be taken if you are on blood thinners like Coumadin or aspirin. Like vitamin C, there is not enough data to support supplementation with large doses of vitamin E.

Alpha Lipoic Acid

Alpha lipoic acid is an antioxidant that works as a cofactor in several biologic reactions in the body. It is commercially available as a dietary supplement and found in some foods, such as liver, spinach, broccoli, and brewer's yeast.

ALPHA LIPOIC ACID AND DIABETES

Alpha lipoic acid has been used in Europe for many years to treat the symptoms of diabetic neuropathy, a common complication of diabetes. Recently, investigators reviewed well-designed studies on alpha lipoic acid that were published between 1966 to 2005 to ascertain whether the nutrient could truly improve the symptoms of diabetic neuropathy in type 1 and type 2 diabetes, or improve blood sugar control. After analyzing these studies, the investigators suggested that alpha lipoic acid could improve symptoms, but only when administered via injections over a three-week period, and not necessarily when taken orally. Also, the article pointed out that alpha lipoic acid does not appear to affect blood sugar control.

PRECAUTIONS

Based on current research, taking alpha lipoic acid as a supplement by mouth does not appear to have benefits for people with diabetes.

Coenzyme Q_{10}

Coenzyme Q_{10} (CoQ_{10}) is a substance produced by the body and felt to be necessary for the basic functioning of cells. Reportedly, CoQ_{10} levels decline with age and are low in patients with chronic diseases involving the heart, muscular dystrophies, Parkinson's disease, cancer, diabetes, and HIV/AIDS. Some prescription drugs may also lower CoQ_{10} levels.

CoQ_{10} is available in supplement form, marketed as tablets and capsules. Concentrations of CoQ_{10} in the body can be increased through supplements, but it is unclear whether this is beneficial to your health.

COQ_{10} AND DIABETES

CoQ_{10} has been used, recommended, or studied for numerous conditions, but remains controversial as a treatment. Some studies hint that it reduces blood glucose and improves the body's use of insulin in diabetes. But there is not yet evidence for these effects in type 1 or type 2 diabetes. CoQ_{10} has also been promoted to treat heart disease, but again, the research is inconclusive.

Another claim for CoQ_{10} is that it reduces blood pressure, since low blood levels have been found in people with hypertension. However, it is unclear whether a CoQ_{10} deficiency actually causes high blood pressure. Some preliminary research suggests that CoQ_{10} may produce small decreases in blood pressure (systolic and, possibly, diastolic).

PRECAUTIONS

There have been a number of serious reported side effects with CoQ_{10} use. Reactions can include nausea, vomiting, stomach upset, heartburn, diarrhea, loss of appetite, and fatigue, among others. We need well-designed, long-term research before a recommendation to supplement with CoQ_{10} can be made.

Botanical Extracts

To date, more than four hundred botanical (plant) treatments for diabetes have been reported, although only a handful have undergone rigorous scientific and medical testing to assess their effectiveness. The use of plants and plant compounds to heal is a form of medicine that has been around for thousands of years—and is still used for about 80 percent of the world's population, particularly in Asia and Europe. Many modern pharmaceutical drugs are derived from herbs, including aspirin (from white willow bark); the heart medication digitalis (foxglove); and the cancer treatment Taxol (Pacific yew tree). Even the blood sugar–lowering drug metformin is derived from galegine, which is naturally found in the herb goat's rue. Today, pharmaceutical companies evaluate plants from around the world to find new compounds that might be proved as remedies and profitably mass marketed. And the World Health Organization Expert Committee on diabetes has recommended that traditional medicinal herbs be further investigated. What follows is a look at some of the most studied and commonly used antidiabetic botanicals. They are also rated as "can't yet be recommended" because we need more data on their effectiveness.

Bitter Melon *(Momordica charantia)*

TRADITIONAL USE
Cultivated in Asia, Africa, and South America, bitter melon has been widely used in folk medicine as a remedy for diabetes. It contains a polypeptide (a string of two or more amino acids) that is similar in structure to bovine insulin.

HOW IT MAY WORK
In four clinical trials conducted with bitter melon juice, fruit, and dried powder, the herb has shown a moderate blood sugar–lowering effect. However, these studies were small and not randomized or double-blinded, and of dubious value.

PRECAUTIONS
The major side effect of bitter melon appears to be gastrointestinal discomfort. A syndrome called favism, a type of anemia, has occurred in people taking bitter melon. It is characterized by headache, fever, abdominal pain, and coma. Currently, due to the inconsistencies in research findings, bitter melon supplements cannot be recommended to treat abnormal levels of blood glucose.

Fenugreek *(Trigonella foenum-graecum)*

TRADITIONAL USE

A member of the pea family, fenugreek is a traditional diabetes remedy that has been used in India for nearly five thousand years. Additionally, it has been widely cultivated in other parts of the world for the treatment of diabetes.

HOW IT MAY WORK

The active ingredients in the defatted portion of the seeds contain compounds called saponins, alkaloids, coumarins, and 4-hydroxyisoleucine, considered to be the main active compound in the herb. This compound reportedly has an insulin-like effect. In rat studies, it has reduced glucose and insulin levels and improved glucose tolerance.

Human studies of fenugreek report reductions in total cholesterol, LDL ("bad" cholesterol), and triglyceride levels, in type 2 diabetics who consumed 25 grams of fenugreek a day. In another study in people with type 2 diabetes, fasting and post-meal blood glucose levels were reduced. To date, however, these trials involved only a small number of subjects and are thus inconclusive.

PRECAUTIONS

Common side effects of supplementing with fenugreek are diarrhea and gas. In addition, this herb may absorb oral medications, so be careful combining it with prescription medicine. Further, fenugreek has the potential to thin your blood due to the coumarins in the plant. Despite the few small studies that have found that fenugreek may help lower blood sugar levels in people with diabetes, there is not enough scientific evidence to support the use of fenugreek.

Gymnema Sylvestre

TRADITIONAL USE

Gymnema sylvestre is an herb derived from the leaves of a tree native to Africa and India. The herb may reduce the desire for sugar by blocking your taste for sweets. It has long been used in India to treat diabetes.

HOW IT MAY WORK

Compounds in the plant are believed to improve blood sugar uptake in the tissues, increase insulin secretion, and increase the number of cells in the pancreas that make insulin.

The truth is, there has been limited research conducted on gymnema sylvestre. A few studies suggest that gymnema sylvestre may decrease fasting glucose and A1c, lower insulin requirements in type 1 diabetes, and reduce the dosage of oral diabetes medications taken by patients with type 2 diabetes.

The problem with these studies, however, is that they are not double-blind or placebo-controlled studies, so it's really difficult to pinpoint a true positive effect without more stringent research.

PRECAUTIONS

Based on the fact that definitive studies have not been done, I can't recommend supplementation with this botanical.

Ivy Gourd *(Coccinia grandis)*

TRADITIONAL USE

Ivy gourd is a creeping plant that grows wild in many parts of India, as well as in tropical areas like Hawaii. It is used in Ayurvedic medicine to treat sugar in the urine, often a symptom of abnormally elevated blood sugar. Ayurvedic medicine is a traditional East Indian healing system. The parts of the herb used in diabetes treatment are the leaves, but the primary use of ivy gourd is culinary, and it is considered a vegetable.

HOW IT MAY WORK

Although this herb has a long history of use, it has not been well researched. Some say that active compounds in the plant may mimic the action of insulin, and may suppress the activity of certain enzymes involved in glucose production.

One double-blind, placebo-controlled study demonstrated that in type 2 diabetics, ivy gourd improved glucose tolerance over six weeks of treatment. Of sixteen patients who received the herbal preparation, ten showed improvement, while no one in the placebo group improved. In one controlled clinical trial of seventy people, the use of dried herb pellets for twelve weeks was suggested to be as effective as treatment with chlorpropamide (an oral blood sugar–lowering drug) for reducing blood glucose levels.

PRECAUTIONS
In the few clinical studies that have been conducted on ivy gourd, no adverse effects were reported. This herb may have potential, but warrants further testing with more stringent design and larger numbers of subjects. I cannot recommend supplementation with ivy gourd until there is more definitive data regarding its effectiveness.

Nopal or Prickly Pear Cactus (Opuntia streptacantha)

TRADITIONAL USE
Prickly pear cactus, as it is known in the United States, is commonly used by people of Mexican descent for glucose control. This plant is cultivated as both a vegetable, called nopal, and a red egg-shaped fruit called tuna. Nopal is a part of soups, salads, sandwiches, and blended in drinks in the traditional Mexican diet.

HOW IT MAY WORK
Prickly pear cactus is very high in soluble fiber, particularly pectin. This may be the most likely reason why it may regulate blood glucose. Other mechanisms of action may be at work too.

In animal studies, prickly pear decreases post-meal levels of glucose and A1c. Two controlled short-term studies of fourteen and twenty-two human subjects, respectively, reported decreased fasting glucose and insulin levels in patients with type 2 diabetes after they took a single dose (500 grams of broiled or grilled nopal stems).

PRECAUTIONS
With the exception of mild gastrointestinal upset, prickly pear cactus in the reported studies appeared to be well tolerated. Even so, longer-term clinical trials are needed to verify if any sustained benefits in the treatment of diabetes are noted. Thus, I can't recommend its use until definitive and carefully controlled studies are conducted.

Ginseng

Used in traditional Chinese medicine for thousands of years, ginseng comes in a number of plant species. These include Chinese or Korean ginseng (*Panax ginseng*), Siberian ginseng (*Eleutherococcus senticosus*), American ginseng (*Panax quiquefolius*), and Japanese ginseng (*Panax japonicus*). Ginseng species are often touted for their "cure-all" properties, including boosting the immune system and increasing stamina, concentration, longevity, and overall well-being.

HOW IT MAY WORK

Researchers believe that the effectiveness of ginseng to improve glucose may stem from compounds in the plant called ginsenosides. Reportedly, these compounds have various effects in the body, including decreasing the rate of carbohydrate absorption into the liver's bloodstream, increasing blood sugar transport and uptake, increasing storage of blood sugar, and increasing insulin secretion.

Most clinical trials have used American ginseng to test the herb's effect on patients with type 2 diabetes. Two longer-term trials administered American ginseng for eight weeks in one study with thirty-six subjects and the other with twenty-four subjects. Both studies reported decreases in fasting blood glucose and A1c. Three other short-term metabolic trials in healthy volunteers also found decreases in glucose after meals.

PRECAUTIONS

There are known side effects of large doses and long-term use: diarrhea, insomnia, nervousness, nausea, and vomiting. Although the available evidence for American ginseng in diabetes suggests a possible hypoglycemic effect, the trials are small and longer-term studies are clearly needed. Thus, I can't make any firm recommendation for its use at this time.

Aloe Vera

TRADITIONAL USE

The sap, or gel, from the leaves of this plant is used topically—to take care of dermatitis and burns (including sunburn), and to enhance wound healing.

Taken internally, aloe juice has been used widely in India and on the Arabian peninsula to treat diabetes.

HOW IT MAY WORK

Aloe contains glucomannan, a fiber that reportedly can drive down blood sugar and make cells more sensitive to insulin. Two nonrandomized clinical trials that studied forty subjects in one study and seventy-six in another reported improved fasting blood glucose with six weeks after using juice made from aloe gel. Also, there is a case report of five people with type 2 diabetes who experienced decreases in fasting blood glucose as well as A1c after supplementing with aloe vera. No adverse effects were reported in these trials. Animal studies looking into its use in diabetes have been mixed.

PRECAUTIONS

Aloe vera should not be taken if you have any sort of intestinal condition, such as Crohn's disease, ulcerative colitis, inflammation in the abdominal area, or any intestinal disorder. The preliminary data suggests a possible effect of aloe vera in glycemic control; however, further information is needed and firm recommendations on its use cannot be made at this time.

Russian Tarragon *(Artemisia dracunculus)*

TRADITIONAL USE

A common medicinal and culinary herb with centuries of use, Russian tarragon is a close relative of the French or cooking tarragon. Even though it goes by the same botanical name (*Artemisia dracunculus*), it is a different strain altogether. In contrast to the aromatic anise flavor of true tarragon, its Russian cousin has a bland, grassy flavor. An extract of Russian tarragon called Tarralin is being investigated for its ability to reduce glucose concentrations in the blood.

HOW IT MAY WORK

Tarralin may work by blocking an enzyme involved in gluconeogenesis, the body's way of creating glucose from the breakdown of proteins in the liver and by improving insulin efficiency. To date, Tarralin's effectiveness has been reported only in animal studies, but human studies are ongoing. In a study I conducted, my colleagues and I found that the extract lowered blood glucose levels in genetically diabetic mice by 24 percent, relative to control animals. In comparison, treatment with the known antidiabetic drugs troglitazone and metformin decreased blood glucose concentrations by 28 percent, and 41 percent, respectively. Blood insulin concentrations were reduced in the genetically diabetic mice by 33 percent with Tarralin; 48 percent with troglitazone; and 52 percent with metformin.

Another study assessed whether Tarralin had any toxic effects in laboratory mice. The animals were given various doses of the extract over the ninety day period, and no toxic effects were found. The researchers concluded that Tarralin appears to be safe and nontoxic based on this experiment.

PRECAUTIONS

Tarralin is a botanical just beginning to be investigated in humans, so we don't yet know what its effects are. Until human testing is completed, recommendations can't be made at this time.

Garlic *(Allium sativum)*

TRADITIONAL USES

For centuries, garlic has been used as a medicinal herb by the ancient Sumerians, Egyptians, Greeks, Chinese, Indians, and later the Italians and English to treat intestinal disorders, flatulence, worms, respiratory infections, skin diseases, wounds, symptoms of aging, and many other ailments. Through the Middle Ages into World War II, garlic was used to treat wounds. It was ground up or sliced and applied directly to wounds to halt the spread of infections. More recently, garlic has been touted as a way to prevent and treat cardiovascular disease and diabetes.

HOW IT MAY WORK

To date, there are more than three thousand publications from all over the world that have confirmed the recognized health benefits of garlic. Garlic is packed with numerous compounds, including antioxidants and allicins that have potential healing effects. For example, allicins may increase the secretion or slow the degradation of insulin, increase enzyme activity, and improve glucose storage ability in the body.

Favorable experimental and clinical effects of garlic preparations (including garlic extract) suggest that the sulfides, one of its chemicals, can reduce cholesterol and may make the blood less sticky. As for diabetes, there are few rigorous studies that have been conducted on garlic, and the findings are conflicting.

PRECAUTIONS

Garlic is generally safe for most adults. However, it reportedly interacts with various types of drugs, including blood thinners. The jury is still out on garlic's role in treating diabetes, and more studies are needed to support whether there is any benefit from garlic for diabetes.

Other Adjunctive Treatments for Diabetes to Consider

Acupuncture

One of the main forms of treatment in traditional Chinese medicine, acupuncture is a procedure in which a practitioner inserts sharp, thin needles into designated points on the skin. This process is believed to adjust and channel the body's energy flow into healthier patterns, and is used to treat a wide variety of illnesses and health conditions. Some Western physicians feel that acupuncture also triggers the release of endorphins, the body's natural painkillers, and thus offers relief from chronic pain. Acupuncture, for example, has been promoted as being effective for people with diabetic neuropathy, the painful nerve damage of diabetes.

If you are interested in trying acupuncture for pain relief of diabetic neuropathy, I suggest you do your homework first and read about all the latest findings to date. It is easy to do by simply visiting a Web site set up by the National Institutes of Health: http://nccam.nih.gov/health/acupuncture. On this site, you'll find the latest studies and recommendations.

Mind-Body Medicine: Biofeedback and Meditation

Biofeedback and meditation are now considered as part of a larger approach of alternative medicine that is referred to as mind-body medicine. As defined by the National Center for Complementary and Alternative Medicine, mind-body medicine typically focuses on intervention strategies that are thought to promote health, such as relaxation, hypnosis, visual imagery, meditation, yoga, biofeedback, tai chi, qi gong, cognitive behavioral therapies, group support, autogenic training, and spirituality. Information on these approaches can be found on the Web site of the National Institutes of Health: http://nccam .nih.gov/health/backgrounds/mindbody.htm.

There has been evidence in support of use of these approaches. For example, in a study at the Medical University of Ohio in 2005, patients with type 2 diabetes were randomized to either ten sessions of biofeedback and relaxation or three sessions of education. All sessions were individual. A total of thirty-nine participants were enrolled, and thirty completed the three-month study. Average blood glucose, A1c, forehead muscle tension, and peripheral skin temperature were assessed, and inventories measuring depression and anxiety were taken prior to, and after completion of the study. Remarkably, biofeedback and relaxation significantly decreased blood sugar, A1c, and muscle tension, compared with the control group. At three-month follow-up, the treatment group continued to demonstrate lower blood glucose and A1c. Both groups decreased their scores on the depression and anxiety inventories.

Meditation, if practiced correctly, appears to be an effective stress reliever. Stress is a part of life, but if you have diabetes, it presents two problems. First, the direct effect of stress on your body raises your blood glucose levels, and second, stress makes you more vulnerable to poor self-care, such as overeating or sitting on the couch and watching TV instead of exercising. Can meditation, a practice that has its origins in civilizations of ancient Africa, Japan, and India, work for you? Research has also suggested that practicing meditation regularly can help you reduce your body's responses to stress by normalizing your blood pressure, slowing your heart rate, and lowering your blood glucose levels. Meditation for health purposes is also being investigated for its effectiveness. To get information on the specifics and benefits of meditation, visit the NIH Web site: http://nccam.nih.gov/health/meditation.

In diabetes, as in many other diseases, it is very important not to substitute proven conventional medical therapy with an alternative therapy. The conventional treatment of diabetes absolutely requires nutrition therapy, exercise, and oral glucose-lowering drugs and/or insulin. This strategy has proven effective to control blood glucose in rigorous studies. And if you have type 1 diabetes, you must take insulin. Be encouraged, too, that so much research is now being devoted to investigating natural supplements, therapies, and other treatments for diabetes. This work adds to the many exciting treatments now available to help you better control your blood sugar and improve your quality of life.

Exercising Your Options

EXERCISE—I KNOW IT *IS* A WONDER worker. Over the last decade, we doctors have increasingly pushed it as one of the best ways to help control type 2 diabetes and improve quality of life for people with type 1 diabetes. Along with nutrition and effective medication, physical activity can help you reduce risk factors for major diseases such as heart disease and stroke, and generally feel better, physically and mentally. And you don't have to spend lots of time working up a sweat either. Nor do you have to follow a structured routine in a gym with fancy equipment. Even if you start with nothing more than a short walk, that's the straightest path to better health.

Mark is a motivating example of what I'm talking about. Mark was diagnosed with type 2 diabetes and had a history of heart disease in his family. Dealing with the highs and lows of blood sugar was nearly overwhelming, and he had only marginal success in controlling it, even while taking an oral diabetes medication. His doctor told him that tighter diabetes control would greatly help him improve his blood sugar control and possibly prevent complications such as heart disease, since his total cholesterol and triglycerides were too high and he needed to lose some weight. Adding some exercise into his treatment plan was recommended. Since Mark wasn't much of an exerciser, his doctor wisely suggested that he find a way to sneak exercise into his life, without making physical activity feel too structured.

"So I began walking to work a few days a week, and walking home," Mark says. "Diet-wise, I started including more unprocessed foods at each meal. I balance the carbs with lean protein. I don't worry too much about fats; I just try to watch them." The results of these decisions have been positive, though not unpredictable when you make permanent changes like Mark did. Mark's total cholesterol dropped from 260 to 170; his triglycerides to 110, from a whopping 375. His weight is down twenty pounds, and his doctor now says Mark should live a long, healthy life if he keeps his diabetes-controlled lifestyle in tact. As Mark ultimately learned, the list of reasons for becoming more active in your life is a long one.

Exercise Helps in the Prevention of Type 2 Diabetes

The Diabetes Prevention Program (DPP), a study I mentioned previously, conclusively showed that people with prediabetes can prevent the development of type 2 diabetes by increasing their level of physical activity and making changes in their diet. They may even be able to return their blood glucose levels within a normal range. While the DPP also showed that some medications may delay the development of diabetes, diet and exercise worked even better. Just thirty minutes a day of moderate physical activity, coupled with a 5 to 10 percent reduction in body weight, produced a 58 percent reduction in diabetes. If you are overweight and your body has already started having trouble metabolizing glucose—in other words, you're prediabetic—then exercise is a must.

Exercise Helps Reduce Blood Levels of Glucose

In a number of studies, lifestyle changes that included exercise were shown to be effective in improving glycemic control, as indicated by the main measure of control: A1c levels. How exactly does exercise do this? It starts in your muscles. Muscles require a constant supply of usable fuel when you exercise. This fuel comes from glucose in your blood and from glycogen, the storage form of glucose in your muscles and liver. As you keep exercising, more glycogen is used up. To compensate, your liver manufactures additional glucose to provide continuous energy. Eventually, glucose stores are reduced, and your body draws from fat for fuel—which is advantageous if you're overweight. Also, contracting your muscles stimulates the movement of glucose into cells. Less insulin is thus required to usher glucose into muscle cells. The bottom line? Exercise affects the very thing you need to control, your blood sugar levels.

I often observe this in my patients. Some time ago, I diagnosed Larry with type 2 diabetes. The thirty-two-year-old insurance agent had gained fifteen pounds over the past five years and had not seen a doctor for several years. Once he came to our clinic, his initial glucose at the time of diagnosis was 165 mg/dl and on repeat was 159 mg/dl. I placed him on metformin and increased his dose 2 grams a day. Additionally, he changed his eating habits and had lost about seven pounds, a weight loss he maintained for six months. His A1c levels were 6.5 percent at that time.

Larry was motivated to completely control blood sugar to normal by becoming more active. I suggested a walking program initially. It was doable, and Larry quickly was able to incorporate three miles of walking a day, four to five days a week. "It became so easy that I would walk faster, then I began to slowly run. Over time, I was running the entire two to three miles and I continue this three to four times a week."

Over several months, Larry lost another five pounds and his A1c level was reduced to 5.9 percent. By maintaining a reduced caloric level and burning more calories through exercise, he was able to lose the rest of his fifteen pounds.

Exercise May Help Reduce the Need for Diabetes Medication

Because exercise makes your blood glucose levels drop, you may need a lower dose of diabetes medication if you have type 2 diabetes. Or in some instances, you may be able to go off pills altogether. Additionally, people with type 1 diabetes, whose bodies don't produce insulin, may find they require a lower dose of insulin after they start exercising on a regular basis.

Exercise Burns Fat and Helps to Control Your Weight

Exercise is a fat burner. Not only does it use up calories, but it also boosts your metabolic rate for hours afterward to help you drop pounds. What's more, it helps you reduce the abdominal fat that is associated with metabolic syndrome and diabetes. And, you're more likely to maintain your weight loss if you make exercise a habit. A lot of people, though, try to lose weight by just dieting—without exercise. Some of your weight loss, unfortunately, will come from muscle tissue, rather than from fat. That's problematic for a couple of reasons. You lose the tissue that gives your body shape and tone and is the major tissue that burns calories. Ideally, you'll want to combine exercise with diet, and the goal would be to lose the pounds from your fat stores more than from your muscles.

Exercise Helps Reduce Cardiovascular Risk

Heart disease is the No. 1 killer of men and women in this country, but it is a particularly ominous risk for people with type 1 or type 2 diabetes. Fortunately, exercise protects you against heart disease—in several ways. Aerobic exercise such as walking, cycling, or jogging improves the efficiency of your heart so that it can pump more blood with each beat. Better circulatory health is important, since many people with diabetes often develop blood vessel problems that lead to very serious complications. Exercise helps reduce your blood pressure. As important, several of these factors are interrelated. For example, when you lower your high blood pressure, your risk for heart disease, stroke, and kidney disease also falls. Another example is that exercise favorably alters your blood lipid profiles. These profiles include measurements of total cholesterol, HDL ("good" cholesterol), LDL ("bad" cholesterol), and triglycerides, all factors that reduce the risk of plaque buildup in the coronary arteries that surround the heart.

Exercise Improves Quality of Life
in Type 1 Diabetes

If you have type 1 diabetes, exercise may not always be effective in helping you improve your blood sugar control, according to several studies that measured A1c in type 1 diabetics. That's not altogether negative news, however. These studies did show that exercise produced valuable benefits, such as reduction of cardiovascular risk factors, increased endurance, better weight control, and an overall feeling of well-being.

So there you have it—exercise is a powerful tool in the fight to control your diabetes and improve your quality of life. Having diabetes provides compelling reasons to begin an exercise program and to stick with it. If physical activity has not been a part of your life, now is the time to get moving.

Preparing for Exercise

Whether you have prediabetes or full-blown diabetes, there are important steps to take prior to starting or resuming an exercise program. These steps will help you get ready:

TALK TO YOUR DOCTOR.

Because diabetes puts you at high risk for heart disease, it is very important that before starting an exercise program, you undergo a detailed medical evaluation. Although you may not have been diagnosed with heart problems, you may have underlying abnormalities in your blood vessels already. Let your doctor know your intention to become more active, so that he or she can clear you to do so. Part of this evaluation may include an exercise test with electrocardiogram (ECG) monitoring to see how your heart reacts to exercise. Your doctor may suggest a heart imaging test at the stress test to better assess your condition.

You must definitely talk to your doctor about exercising if: you are over the age of thirty-five; you've had diabetes for ten years or longer; you have a history of heart disease or high blood pressure; you're overweight; or you're taking medication. During your examination, your doctor looks for any signs of large or small blood vessel damage, nerve damage, and evidence of cardiovascular risk factors such as smoking that may affect your exercise performance and health. If the tests show signs of disease, talk to your doctor about which physical activities will help you, but without making your condition worse.

CHOOSE AN APPROPRIATE FORM OF EXERCISE.

The best exercise for you is something you enjoy doing, because if you like it, you're more likely to stick with it. Also, the type of exercise you do depends very much on the state of your health and diabetic condition. If you have diabetes, but are managing certain complications, there are particular kinds of exercises to avoid since they could aggravate your health. Your exercise choices will depend on the condition of your heart, blood vessels, eyes, kidneys, feet, and nervous system (see the section on page 168 for specifics). What follows is an overview of the various types of exercise to consider, and the benefits of each.

Aerobic Exercise Aerobic exercise consists of rhythmic, repeated, and continuous movements of the same large muscle groups for at least ten minutes at a time. Walking, bicycling, jogging, swimming, water aerobics, and many forms of sports are examples of aerobic exercise. It trains your heart, lungs, and circulatory system to process oxygen and transport it to your muscles more efficiently. It also burns calories and body fat, plus increases your metabolism. Furthermore, it enhances your lung capacity, reduces blood pressure, strengthens your immune system, and lowers stress levels.

Whatever aerobic activity you do, a good rule of thumb is to exercise within your *target heart range*, a zone in which you should be working out in order to most benefit your body. If you're really looking to burn calories, try to maintain a heart range on the higher end of your range. However, what can't be stated enough is that if you have diabetes or underlying heart problems, a target heart range may not be appropriate for you and may actually precipitate further heart problems. Simply put, you may have problems with your heart that will preclude such an activity and heart range. This is why it is so important to first be medically evaluated before you even consider such a vigorous exercise program. However, with that being stated, formulas have been provided that allow you to calculate your *target heart range* if appropriate for your underlying condition:

1. Take your *resting heart rate* first thing in the morning; count the number of beats in one minute (or, alternatively, the number of beats in thirty

seconds and multiply by 2). To find your heart rate, take your pulse at the radial artery in either wrist.

2. Calculate your *maximum heart rate* by subtracting your age from 220. You'll need to determine the heart rate range that you should be working at by calculating your maximum heart rate. Maximum heart rate equals the number of times your heart would beat in a minute if you were running as fast as you possibly could.

3. Subtract your resting heart rate from your maximum heart rate to determine your *heart rate reserve*.

4. Multiply your *heart rate reserve* by 0.5 and 0.7 to determine the range of your heart rate reserve. When added to your resting heart rate, this yields the *target heart range* for your aerobic workout.

For example, let's say you're forty-five years old, with a *resting heart rate* of seventy beats per minute. Your *maximum heart rate* is 220−45=175. Your *heart rate reserve* is 175−70=105. The *range* of your heart rate reserve is from 105 × 0.5 = 53 to 105× 0.7 = 74. Your *target range* for your workout out is from 53 + 70 = 123 to 74 + 70 = 144, or 123 − 144.

Consider the use of a heart rate monitor to help keep yourself in your target range while exercising aerobically. This tool will tell you exactly what your heart rate is as you're exercising. Some exercise equipment, such as treadmills, comes with built-in monitors. But there are wristwatch varieties you can use too.

Another gadget worth your investment is a pedometer. This device, which clips to your waistband or clothes, automatically counts your steps as you go through your day. Wear it for a couple of days to see how many steps you take daily. Once you know how many steps you average daily, you're ready to set some targets. Aim to add two thousand more steps every day until you hit ten thousand or more (which is equivalent to approximately five miles, burns an extra 400 to 500 calories a day, and is the number many experts recommend for good health). As a handy frame of reference, here is how your daily steps stack up in terms of active results:

- Sedentary: Less than 5,000
- Low level of activity: 5,000 to 7,499

- Somewhat active: 7,500 to 9,999
- Active: 10,000 to 12,499
- Highly active: Greater than 12,500

Achieving ten thousand steps or more daily translates into lost pounds too. In one study, four hundred women, ages nineteen to seventy-one, were encouraged to walk ten thousand steps each day for eight weeks and to wear a pedometer while doing so. By the end of the study, nearly half of the women reported losing weight. Those who set daily step goals also said they improved their muscle tone, increased their energy, fit into their clothes better, and felt less stressed out.

Strength Training Strength training consists of activities that use muscular strength to move a weight or work against a resistive load. Examples include weight lifting, or exercises using weight machines, resistance bands, or your body's own weight. These activities develop muscle tissue, and the more muscle you have the better your body can burn fat. This is because muscle is the body's most metabolically active tissue; it is burning calories every moment of the day, even when you are resting or sleeping. Strength training builds bones too, and they become more dense and less prone to osteoporosis and injury. With stronger, better-developed muscles, your joints are better protected from wear and tear. Strength training also improves glucose tolerance and insulin sensitivity, thus allowing you to better control your diabetes.

A word of advice: according to the American Diabetes Association, strength training using weights may be acceptable for younger people with diabetes, but not for older individuals or those with long-standing diabetes. Moderate weight training programs that employ light weights and high repetitions can be used for maintaining or enhancing upper body strength in nearly all patients with diabetes.

If you've never done strength training before, consider exercising with a qualified trainer, if possible, at a gym or facility that can provide assistance.

Mind-Body Exercise Mind-body exercises include yoga, tai chi, or Pilates, which you can do in classes at gyms, health clubs, or wellness centers. Yoga is an ancient Indian discipline that links stretching exercises, breathing, and meditation through the repetition of a series of poses. Tai chi is a slow-motion form of Chinese martial arts designed to increase the "chi," or life energy. Pilates is a muscle-lengthening program developed in Germany in the 1920s. All three are easy to learn; the more you practice, the more adept you become. You may find that mind-body workouts reduce muscular tension, relax your body, and with enhanced flexibility, may protect against injuries. There are even videos available for yoga and other types of exercises that are possible to buy or rent if the cost of going to a health club on a regular basis is not affordable.

Lifestyle Activity If you just don't like formal exercise, here's what I suggest: focus on lifestyle activities. These include walking your dog, doing housework, gardening, playing actively with your kids, dancing—in short, just moving around more as you go about your day. Lifestyle activities pay huge health dividends, according to numerous studies. To begin with, they work wonders when combined with nutrition therapy for management of prediabetes and diabetes. They help tremendously in weight control. Gardening and yardwork, for example, can burn approximately 350 calories an hour; cleaning your house, 250 calories an hour; moving household items around, 500 calories an hour; and dancing, about 300 calories an hour. You can achieve reasonable fitness almost automatically by finding more ways to move your body during the day. And you can even play sports. Many world-class athletes have diabetes, and famous competitors with the condition have included professional tennis players Arthur Ashe and Billy Jean King; some of baseball's all-time greats like Ty Cobb, Jackie Robinson, and Catfish Hunter; and boxers Joe Frazier and Sugar Ray Robinson.

An Exercise Prescription to Prevent Diabetes

Exercise of any kind can lower your risk of getting diabetes. For prevention, you may want to consider some form of strength training in your program. One reason we're seeing this epidemic of type 2 diabetes worldwide is because people are not eating nutritiously, and are becoming more sedentary. When muscles aren't used, their cells become resistant to the insulin that the pancreas secretes. Insulin therefore doesn't do its job. Even a few bouts of strength-building exercise may stimulate muscles to be less resistant to insulin.

There is also some evidence that strength training can reduce abdominal fat. If you carry extra weight around your waist—which has been described as having an apple shape—you're at greater risk of heart disease and diabetes. It has become clear that apple-shaped individuals are prone to metabolic syndrome: they are more likely to be resistant to insulin, have high triglycerides, and have too-low levels of beneficial HDL ("good" cholesterol). They also tend to have high blood pressure. Exercise that incorporates strength training may help reverse these unhealthy characteristics. Aerobic exercise is important too, a great fat burner, and should be included.

Since part of the DPP involved exercise, I want to outline for you what was prescribed in this landmark study on prevention. Here are some key DPP prevention guidelines regarding exercise:

1. Burn up to 700 calories a week.

You easily do this by engaging in only two and a half hours of moderate physical activity a week. This activity could include brisk walking, strength training, or anything you like to do. Work up to this goal *slowly*. It will take about four weeks. Spread the weekly total over three to four days (or more) per week. Only increase a little at a time how often, how hard, and how long you're active.

You *can* find the time to be active. Reserve one block of time every day to be active. When can you set aside twenty to thirty minutes to do an activity you like?

Look for free time (ten to fifteen minutes) during the day. Use the time to be active.

2. Maintain a record of your physical activity.

Keeping track of your activity brings home the need for doing it, plus helps you reach your weekly exercise goals and make progress toward them.

Here is a sample log that you can use to record your progress:

	Kind of Physical Activity	Minutes
Monday	*Walked to the grocery store*	15
Tuesday	*Worked out with weights*	30

(continued)

(continued)

	Kind of Physical Activity	Minutes
Wednesday	Logged 10,000 steps	Throughout the day
Thursday	Attended a yoga class	45
Friday		
Saturday		
Sunday		
Total minutes for the week:		

3. Choose proper footwear.

You don't *need* to buy special shoes if you have shoes now that fit well and support your feet. But here are some pointers if you are planning to buy shoes:

- Look for a good fit. Be sure to tell the salesperson the kind of activity you plan to do. Many shoes are made for a specific activity, such as running or aerobic dancing. They will give you the kind of support needed for that activity. Also, take your old shoes with you to the store. Ask the salesperson to look at the pattern of wear. This can show the kind of support you need. For example, is the back of the shoe worn down unevenly on the bottom (that is, does it slant toward the inside or outside)? If so, you may need extra support for arches or flat feet. Your shoes should match the shape of your foot and the way your feet strike the ground.
- Wear the kind of socks you'll wear when you're active.
- Get the kind of foot support you need. Along with socks, the use of silica gel or air midsoles to prevent blisters and keep your feet dry is important for minimizing trauma to the feet.
- Monitor your feet closely for blisters and other potential damage to your feet, both before and after physical activity.

4. Stay hydrated.

Drinking water is essential, since dehydration can adversely affect your blood glucose levels and heart function. After physical activity, drink additional fluid to compensate for any losses in sweat. Be sure you're well hydrated if exercising in extremely hot or cold environments.

5. Incorporate lifestyle activities into your day.

Make active choices throughout the day. Every minute adds up to a more active you. Use the work sheet below to jot down some ideas.

Inactive Choice (Limit)	Active Choice
When you shop, park your car as close as you can to the entrance to the store.	Park your car farther away and walk.

Other ideas: turn inactive into active time. For example, try cutting your TV time in half. Walk instead. Or be active while you watch TV: ride an exercise bike or lift weights.

6. Warm up before and cool down after every activity.

A standard recommendation for diabetic patients, as for nondiabetic individuals, is that physical activity should include proper warm-up and cooldown periods. A warm-up should consist of five to ten minutes of aerobic activity (walking, cycling, and so forth) at a low-intensity level. Your warm-up session prepares your muscles, heart, and lungs for a progressive increase in exercise intensity. After a short warm-up, gently stretch your muscles for another five to ten minutes, particularly the muscles you'll use during exercise, although warming up all muscle groups is optimal. The active warm-up can take place either before or after stretching. After the activity session, perform a cooldown. The cooldown should last about five to ten minutes and gradually bring your heart rate down to its pre-exercise level. I've included a series of recommended stretches in Appendix B.

7. Listen to your body.

No matter what type of exercise you ultimately do, be alert to any sensations that come up while you're exercising. If you detect any complaint from your body, such as pain or discomfort, identify the origin. Then make small adjustments in your technique or posture and see whether the complaint lessens. Stop exercising if you experience an uncomfortable feeling of pressure, pain, squeezing, or heaviness, particularly in the center of your chest, spread throughout the front of your chest, or radiating to your shoulder(s), arm(s), neck, and back. If it doesn't go away after two to four minutes, go to an emergency room. If it does go away, you will still need to be evaluated by your doctor. It may be a sign of heart disease. Also, be alert to signs such as severe nausea, shortness of breath, sweating, or feeling light-headed. These may or may not be signs of something serious like a heart problem, and you should notify your doctor.

An Exercise Prescription for Managing Diabetes

If you have been diagnosed with diabetes or have complications, you must be exceedingly careful when exercising. You will probably need to emphasize low-intensity exercise such as walking, swimming, aquatic exercise, stationary cycling, stretching, yoga, Pilates, any non-weight-bearing exercise, or non-jarring forms of aerobics. These forms of exercise will not aggravate existing complications, but will help you get healthier, control your weight, and stay in shape.

Exercise and Diabetes Complications

Depending on recommendations from your physician, try to do at least 150 to 180 minutes a week of low-intensity aerobic physical activity. With complications, exercise choice is the most critical factor, since diabetic complications rule out certain forms of physical activity. The sections below give recommendations for exercise based on your physical condition.

Retinopathy

If you have been diagnosed with retinopathy, strenuous exercise may cause hemorrhaging or a retinal detachment. Here are important guidelines:

Avoid these:
* Any form of strength training
* High-impact aerobic exercise such as running, jogging, vigorous aerobic dance classes, or any type of jarring activity

- Exercise with jarring movements such as mountain biking, skydiving, gymnastics, martial arts, boxing, and so forth
- Any activity or exercise in which your face is placed in the head-down position
- Contact sports like basketball or football

Try these:
- Riding a stationary bike
- Taking a brisk walk on a treadmill
- Rowing at an easy pace on a rowing machine
- Dancing with a partner who can guide you
- Participating in water exercises or aqua aerobics
- Swimming laps, and guiding yourself by touching the pool's lane ropes if your vision is impaired

Nephropathy

The key here is to avoid activities that are high intensity (like those listed above under retinopathy), since they can increase your blood pressure. If your workout feels too hard, it probably is. You can still perform strength training, but use light weights and higher repetitions. Never strain when lifting weights.

Try these:
- Riding a stationary bike
- Taking a brisk walk on a treadmill
- Rowing at an easy pace on a rowing machine
- Participating in water exercises or aqua aerobics
- Swimming

Nerve Damage in the Limbs

If you have nerve damage to your hands, legs, or feet, you may feel pain, tingling, or numbness in those areas. Exercise won't cure the problem, but it can help by building your strength, increasing flexibility, and encouraging blood flow to those damaged areas. If you combine regular exercise with good blood glucose control, you may be able to relieve some of the pain.

Avoid these:

- Jogging
- Prolonged walking
- Treadmill exercise
- Step aerobics

Good choices if you have nerve damage in your legs or feet are activities that don't put a lot of stress on your legs, feet, or nearby joints.

Try these:

- Bicycling
- Stationary cycling
- Swimming
- Aqua aerobics
- Light rowing on a rowing machine

If pushing with your feet on a bicycle doesn't feel good or is not safe, you can try a special machine in which you can pedal with your arms.

Be sure to take good care of your feet and check them periodically. Wear shoes such as water socks while you are in the water or walking around the pool and locker room area. If you have an open wound, do not use the pool until it heals.

Blood Vessel Damage

Some people with diabetes have a condition known as intermittent claudication, in which the blood vessels in the legs close up and circulation to the muscles is sluggish. The main symptom of intermittent claudication is an aching pain in your legs when you walk. Exercise helps increase blood flow in the legs. A good choice is interval walking, in which you alternate resting and walking short distances to avoid pain and fatigue. Cycling and swimming are also good options.

Autonomic Neuropathy

With autonomic neuropathy, avoid activities that require quick changes in body position, such as basketball, volleyball, racquet sports, and other such sports. You may also have problems with low blood pressure, which can make you faint. Do not exercise at high intensity. More suitable exercise choices include recumbent stationary cycling (using a special kind of bike that allows you to stretch your legs out in front to pedal) and aqua aerobics.

Heart Disease and High Blood Pressure

If you have heart disease or high blood pressure, you can still benefit from regular exercise, particularly walking. But I recommend that you work out a program with your doctor and exercise specialist. In fact, your doctor may refer you to a cardiac rehabilitation program. This is a medically supervised program that tests your fitness level and makes specific exercise suggestions for you. When you start to exercise in such a program, you can build your confidence and abilities in a safe environment.

Organ Transplantation

Following an organ transplant, when you are well enough, try a program of aerobic and strength training exercises. The reason is, organ transplantation usually leads to weight gain for people with diabetes; this is a side effect of antirejection drugs. Although they help your body accept the new organ, these drugs can lead to weight gain and muscle wasting. You need to go slowly, however. Discuss your exercise program with your diabetes care team and an exercise specialist.

Amputation and Limited Mobility

If you have limited mobility from diabetes or other health problems (such as arthritis), some good exercise choices might be water exercise or chair aerobics. Often, there are special classes available for all of these types of classes. Staying with regular exercise can help you keep the mobility you have. Or you may have had a foot or leg amputation. If your feet can't hold your body weight, try riding a stationary bike, doing chair exercises, or some form of water exercise. You will be surprised how much exercise can help improve your strength and flexibility. Discuss your options with your doctor and exercise specialist.

If You Use Insulin: Exercise Guidelines

If you have type 1 diabetes, or type 2 diabetes and are taking insulin, you will need to make adjustments in your insulin if you exercise, since exercise can trigger a drop in glucose levels, during, immediately after, or many hours after physical activity. In order to make these adjustments, you'll need to closely monitor your glucose levels, and use this data to improve your exercise performance and enhance exercise safety.

Here are some general guidelines, including those from the American Diabetes Association, that may prove helpful in regulating the glycemic response to physical activity:

- Always measure your blood glucose before and after exercising.
- Before physical activity: avoid exercising if your fasting glucose levels are greater than 250mg/dl and ketosis is present, and use caution if your glucose levels are greater than 300 mg/dl. Use ketone test strips to check your urine for the presence of ketones.
- Eat some additional carbohydrates if your glucose levels are less than 100 mg/dl—for example, a cup of orange juice or a piece of fruit or bread. Then test fifteen to thirty minutes later. Don't start exercising until your blood glucose rises above 100 mg/dl.
- Have carbohydrates on hand readily during and after physical activity.
- Identify when you need to make changes in insulin or food intake, and learn to recognize how your blood sugar reacts to different types of exercise and exercise intensity.
- Always begin your exercise session at least one hour after your last insulin administration. Avoid exercise during the time of peak insulin action. If you're using short-acting insulins, peak insulin action may be at one hour after administration; therefore, exercise should be delayed even longer.
- If you're using injectable insulin, it is absorbed much more quickly when injected close to muscles that are being exercised. The longer the interval between injecting insulin and exercising, the less important the injection site becomes.
- Have a meal or snack two to three hours before exercise and immediately afterward.
- If you experience symptoms of low blood sugar during exercise, stop immediately and measure your glucose levels. (It is a good idea to exercise with someone who is familiar with signs of low blood sugar in case you need help.) Eat a quick-acting carbohydrate source such as glucose tablets, raisins, or hard sugar candy. Signs of low blood sugar included shak-

iness, hunger, nervousness, fatigue, headache, confusion, dizziness, and rapid heartbeat.

* Wear a diabetes identification tag and carry a cellular phone in case of an emergency.

Staying Motivated

Once you become hooked on exercise, the benefits add up quickly. But gearing up and getting started on an exercise program can be the tough part. Here are some suggestions to help you stick with it and make exercise a permanent part of your diabetes prevention and management plan:

* Think of exercise as a part of your daily routine (like brushing your teeth) and build it into your schedule.

* To prevent boredom from setting in, vary your routine and the type of exercises you do. Alternate aerobic exercise on one day with strength training the next day, for example.

* Choose activities you enjoy and can do with a reasonable amount of skill. What really matters, is that you find an exercise that you like, and that it gets your body moving and your heart pumping.

* Work out with a partner for safety, companionship, encouragement, and accountability.

* Set realistic exercise goals that you can accomplish such as: to complete twenty minutes nonstop on a walk or making it to the gym three times a week.

* Take note of your progress: do your clothes fit better? Do you have more energy? Has your blood sugar control improved? Then reward yourself for sticking to your exercise program. Examples of rewards are a new pair of running shoes, new exercise clothes, a workout bag, a massage, facial, or soak in a hot tub.

* Join a gym that's convenient to your home, one that you pass by nearly every day—perhaps on the road between your home and work. Seeing it regularly will prompt you in there to exercise.

* Join an exercise class if you like the social elements of exercising. The camaraderie you develop with your classmates should be enough to keep you coming back.

- Take an iPod or portable CD player to the gym and listen to music while you walk on the treadmill or pedal on a stationary bike. Associating your workouts with fun music will make the activity more appealing.
- Record your blood glucose levels, the medication you've taken, and the carbohydrates you eat. This information will help you gauge various variables in your program and how they affect your glycemic control.

Getting your mind, body, and spirit in gear for exercise isn't an overnight process, but a daily journey. Start today, and know that you're taking the first and most important steps to looking better, feeling better, and living longer.

Glucose Testing Made Pain-Free and Easy

*

Depending on your specific treatment, you may have to test your blood sugar several times a day. If you do, you'll greatly reduce your odds of developing, or worsening, diabetic complications.

But here's the dilemma most patients have: testing your blood sugar is one of the most dreaded tasks of diabetes management because it traditionally involves having to prick your finger to get a droplet of blood. However, testing your blood sugar has become so much easier and with much less pain, thanks to new technologies. And that is great news. Why? With less pain and less hassle, you're likely to test more frequently, and frequent testing keeps you alert to blood sugar swings. That way, you can stabilize them and ultimately prevent diabetes-related health consequences.

Proof of the power of frequent testing comes from the Diabetes Control and Complications Trial (DCCT) and the United Kingdom Prospective Diabetes Study (UKPDS), both of which I discussed in previous chapters. The

DCCT, conducted from 1983 to 1993 by the National Institute of Diabetes and Digestive and Kidney Diseases, was, at the time, the most comprehensive diabetes study ever. It involved 1,441 volunteers with type 1 diabetes at twenty-nine medical centers across the United States and Canada. This study compared the effects of two treatment regimens—*standard therapy* (typically two shots of insulin a day) and *intensive control*—on the complications of diabetes. Participants in the intensive control part of this study were suggested to test their blood sugar levels *four or more times a day* and took four daily insulin injections or used an insulin pump. They adjusted their insulin dose according to their food intake and exercise, followed a diet and exercise plan, and met with their health-care team monthly. The results: intensive therapy reduced the risk of diabetic nerve damage (neuropathy) by 60 percent, diabetic kidney disease by 50 percent, and diabetic eye disease by 76 percent. Over time, it was shown that the intensive therapy reduced the risk of cardiovascular disease and heart attack by 46 percent and the risk of stroke by 57 percent.

Although the DCCT focused on people with type 1 diabetes, its findings were validated by the UKPDS, which compared conventional (nutritional) and intensive therapy (medications) in more than five thousand newly diagnosed people with type 2 diabetes. The UKPDS confirmed that reducing blood sugar levels dramatically reduces the risk of complications in people with type 2 diabetes. It also found that controlling blood pressure, among those with diabetes whose blood pressure is high, dramatically reduces the risk of diabetes complications—especially including the risk of strokes and the risk of vision damage. Make no mistake: keeping your diabetes under tight control greatly reduces your risk of all the major complications of diabetes, and can help you live a long, healthy, and fulfilling life.

As a clinician working in diabetes care, I strive to help my patients manage their diabetes better, but I'm aware, unfortunately, that many people with diabetes often do not achieve their A1c levels, and instead over time they develop diabetes complications. We've clearly seen through landmark studies like the DCCT and the UKPDS that intensive diabetes control that requires frequent self-monitoring of blood glucose is vital to managing the disease and preventing its complications.

Over the years, doctors have realized that many patients, for the most part, simply don't like finger-stick testing, and the fact that they don't like to test often will interfere in the goal of achieving tighter blood sugar control.

Your provider will alter your medications based on your glucose control. One way your provider assesses your control is to obtain the A1c test as discussed. But, day-to-day management to assess blood glucose is up to you. If the data is not available to your doctor to assess your day-to-day blood glucose, he or she may not be able to change the medication dose, such as insulin, to achieve better daily control.

I know what you're thinking—the idea of testing blood sugar four times a day is initially intimidating—and I understand. But with the introduction of continuous glucose monitoring systems (you'll learn about them here), which are implanted under the skin, this often-dreaded task became doable and in many ways has revolutionized self-care.

For example, a forty-six-year-old patient of mine named Nancy has type 1 diabetes and is on an insulin pump. Although she tested herself at fairly regular intervals, she wasn't consistent enough and had highly variable blood sugar control as a result. She was placed on a continuous glucose monitoring system for three days. This system allowed for a comprehensive profile of her glucose over twenty-four hours.

Of course, from my standpoint as a provider, I got a more complete picture of her glycemic control on a twenty-four-hour basis. With this glucose level information, I could adjust her bolus (meal-related) and basal (between meal) rates to ensure she received precisely the insulin she needs, when she needs it. By getting the proper basal rate and bolus dosing, and thus minimizing the high glucose peaks and the low blood sugar swings, Nancy has felt much better than ever since she started managing her diabetes. She checks her glucose before meals and at bedtime now. As a result of this information and being able to "smooth" out her blood glucose profile, her A1c dropped one full point and continues to go down.

A Prescription for Self-Monitoring of Blood Glucose

One of my most important messages throughout this book, and one that can't be stated or emphasized enough, is that one of the keys to tight glucose control over the long term is to know what your blood glucose control is on a daily basis. This process is referred to as self-monitoring of blood glucose, or SMBG. SMBG gives you valuable information about:

- Where your blood sugar stands, so you know whether it is high or low at that particular time, or even changing such as going rapidly from a high value to a lower value over a specified time. This information helps you prevent emergency situations from developing. That way, you can respond to, and prevent problems such as a low blood sugar from developing.
- The amount of insulin to take. If you take what is known as rapid- or short-acting insulin (see Chapter 11) before meals, your blood sugar test, in addition to the amount of carbohydrates you may eat, can help you determine how much insulin you may need to administer before that meal. In addition, if you take a basal or long-acting insulin, checking your blood glucose at certain times, such as between meals, will help you decide what dose to take.
- The effect of exercise, diet, stress, and being ill on your blood sugar levels.
- Trends in blood sugar that you'll want to report to your physician and diabetes educator.

To really appreciate the value of SMBG, we can adapt the saying that "if you take care of your pennies, the dollars will take care of themselves." Well, it's analogous to home blood glucose monitoring. Generally, the averages of your daily SMBG should correlate well to the A1c test that your physician will obtain to assess your control over two to three months. So, assessing SMBG frequently and averaging the blood glucoses should give you a good idea of the long-range control that will be measured by the A1c test. Specifically, taking care of your glucose on a daily basis will take care of the control you will require over the long term. There are two general ways to monitor: traditional methods and implantable methods.

Traditional Self-Monitoring Systems

A traditional home monitoring system consists of equipment to obtain a blood sample and a glucose meter that reads that blood sample. With most systems, you must prick your finger to draw a tiny blood sample. But now there are systems that let you use sites other than your fingertip, such as your forearm, which may be less painful. Depending on the site you use, you'll prick it with a special lancet, obtain a blood droplet, put the blood on a test strip, and insert the strip into the glucose meter. Alternatively, some of the meters will have you insert the strip in the meter prior to placing the drop of blood. Most glucose meters calculate blood sugar either chemically, by using an enzyme that changes color in the presence of glucose; or electrically, by measuring the current generated by glucose oxidation. The meter displays the results of a blood sugar test within a minute or less after testing.

Several new models can record and store a number of test results. That way, you don't always have to keep a written log. Some of the more sophisticated meters include alarm clocks and can record time, date, insulin, doses, exercise, and food intake (including the grams of carbohydrate you've eaten). In addition, computer programs are available that let you analyze this data and print it out to see trends in your glucose control. Some models can connect to personal computers so you can download the data. You and your doctor will use this record to see how often your blood sugar levels have been within the recommended range, or to decide if a change in medication (insulin or pills) for diabetes is needed.

The New Generation of Glucose Testing

IMPLANTABLE CONTINUOUS GLUCOSE MONITORS

Traditionally, people with diabetes have tested for glucose by pricking a finger with a needle (called a lancet) to draw blood—which can be somewhat painful and is required several times a day. This method of testing has been used for years and is effective as part of an intensive regimen. Monitoring does make tight control of diabetes possible—but only if more people would comply. After all, who really likes the idea of pricking their fingers?

Because of technological advances, we now have new methods of glucose monitoring available. These devices are called implantable continuous glucose monitors, and they're inserted under your skin to give you continuous measurements and readings of your glucose levels. Implantable monitors are truly revolutionizing the management of diabetes care by making glucose monitoring user friendly, painless, and easy. Unfortunately, even today, there are still hurdles to the new technologies including cost and the fact that most still require checking with the traditional meters.

Many different types of implantable continuous glucose monitors are on the market, but they all work in a similar fashion. A small, disposable sensor is inserted under your skin through a tiny flexible probe. This sensor detects changes in glucose levels in the fluid around your cells, and dispatches this information to a beeper-sized box, which stores the results. Several days' worth of data can be stored at a time. Some monitors give an audible glucose report, which is very beneficial if you're visually impaired. Others combine the monitor with a wrist blood pressure monitor—eliminating the need for two separate devices. Both type 1 and type 2 patients can use implantable glucose monitors.

Another advantage of these monitors is that they can give you and your doctor a clearer picture of blood sugar trends throughout the day in order to identify problems and make adjustments to your insulin, meals, or exercise program. The monitors also have alert systems to let you know if your blood glucose is on the way up or down, as well as if it becomes dangerously high or dangerously low.

Currently, three implantable glucose monitors are on the U.S. market. They are the DexCom™ STS™, Guardian® RT, and MiniMed Continuous Glucose Monitoring System, with more on the way. Talk with your doctor about the availability of these products and whether a continuous glucose monitor makes sense for you. Here is a brief look at what is available, as of this writing:

- *The DexCom™ STS™ Continuous Glucose Monitoring System.* This system consists of three components: an implantable sensor, a transmitter, and a receiver. It provides real-time continuous glucose measurements every five minutes for up to three days (seventy-two hours), and has adjustable high and low glucose alerts to notify you when you are outside your target glucose levels. Please be aware, however, that this device is not designed to replace a blood glucose meter, but the DexCom STS System must be used with a blood glucose meter. As such, the DexCom STS Continuous Glucose Monitoring System is indicated for use as an adjunctive device to complement, not replace, information obtained from standard home glucose monitoring devices. Treatment decisions should not be based solely on results from the DexCom STS System. You must confirm with a blood glucose meter before making therapeutic adjustments.
- *The Guardian® RT.* This device has a tiny sensor inserted under your skin using a special insertion device. A small, waterproof transmitter is taped to your skin, so you can wear it all the time. The transmitter uses

wireless technology to send glucose values automatically to a compact monitor. The monitor displays updated glucose readings every five minutes and alarms sound when levels become too high or too low. The monitor can store up to twenty-one days' worth of information that can be downloaded to your computer. The monitor and transmitter aren't physically connected and can even be as far as six feet apart. The manufacturers advise using this system to supplement blood glucose information from standard home blood glucose meters, in which you do a finger prick to obtain a blood sample.

- *MiniMed Continuous Glucose Monitoring System.* This system consists of a small plastic catheter (very small tube) inserted just under the skin. The catheter collects small amounts of liquid that are passed through a sensor to measure the amount of glucose present. It takes a blood glucose measurement every five minutes throughout the day and night, for up to three days. Currently, the results are not viewable instantly, but have to be downloaded later to a computer. Your physician may suggest that you use this system for a three-day period so that he or she can assess swings in your blood sugar and allow him or her the ability to match insulin dosing with peaks and troughs in your profile.

- *Noninvasive Monitors.* "Noninvasive monitoring" means checking blood glucose levels without having to puncture your skin for a blood sample. An example is the GlucoWatch G2 Biographer, which is worn on your arm like a wristwatch. It draws body fluid from your skin using small electric currents and can provide six measurements per hour for thirteen hours. The GlucoWatch then displays the results. It is useful for detecting and evaluating episodes of hyperglycemia and hypoglycemia. However, the G2 Biographer is intended to supplement, not replace, conventional blood glucose monitoring, and the manufacturer recommends that you confirm the results with a standard glucose meter and finger stick testing.

USING LASERS TO OBTAIN A BLOOD SAMPLE

Another less painful alternative to finger stick testing is the use of a battery-operated laser tool, rather than a lancet. Called Lasette Plus, this device vaporizes a tiny hole in your fingertip to create the small opening needed to obtain the blood drop. You would then use your test strips and glucose meter as normal. There are different power adjustments you can try to make it less painful for you. Using a laser device may help reduce tissue trauma and residual soreness that you might otherwise experience with a lancet.

Your Target Range What blood glucose level should you be aiming for when you test? As a frame of reference, normal blood sugar level for someone without diabetes is suggested to be less than 100 mg/dl fasting and less than 120 mg/dl two hours after a meal. Your doctor and diabetes educator may set a different target range for you, and you should try to stay within that range. The American Diabetes Association suggests the following targets:

A1c	Less than 7.0%
Preprandial plasma glucose (before a meal)	90 to 130 mg/dl
Postprandial plasma glucose (after a meal)	Less than 180 mg/dl

Of course, if you have diabetes and vascular disease or multiple cardiovascular risk factors, including high blood pressure, high cholesterol, obesity, and smoking, your goal may be adjusted. This suggested adjustment came about as a result of the Action to Control Cardiovascular Risk in Diabetes (ACCORD) study. Some 10,251 participants were in groups receiving three types of treatment: intensive lowering of blood sugar, lowering blood pressure, or reducing cholesterol. Suprisingly, the study found that trying to hit a target blood sugar goal of an A1c of less than 6 percent, which is similar to blood sugar levels in adults without diabetes, was harmful and could even increase the risk of cardiovascular events in high-risk patients. As of yet, there is no explanation as to why.

Don't expect to be perfect 100 percent of the time. That's virtually impossible—everyone has occasional slips—but a goal is to have the averages of the values stay within your range most of the time. These averages should relate to the long-term control test, the A1c. Your glucose meter is another important tool that will help you stay on the road to good health.

Maintaining Your Equipment Blood sugar testing equipment, like any other equipment, requires proper care and maintenance to ensure that you get accurate results. It's important to follow these procedures to keep your equipment in good working order:

- Read carefully, and follow, the manufacturer's instructions.
- Try not to drop or bump your meter.
- Do not store your meter in a very hot or very cold place.
- Clean your meter regularly, and change the batteries as instructed. If you think a test result from your meter is different from what you expected, repeat the test. If you get similar results with the second test, you may need to talk with your health professional about what to do next.
- Perform quality-control checks to make sure that your home glucose testing is accurate and reliable, either with a control solution or using electronic controls. Essentially, when you run a quality-control test, you substitute the test solution for blood. If the results of your test match the values given in the quality-control solution labeling, you can be assured the entire system (meter and test strip) is working properly. If the results are not correct, the system may not be accurate, and you'll need to contact the manufacturer for advice. Some glucose meters also use electronic controls to make sure the meter is working properly. With this method, you insert a test cartridge or a special "control" test strip in the meter and a signal will appear to indicate whether the meter is working properly.
- In addition, it is always a good idea to check the accuracy of your glucose meter at the same time your blood sugar is tested at your doctor's office or lab.
- Do not share lancets, either, or throw them into the household trash. A used lancet might accidentally puncture someone. A very good suggestion is that you dispose of your used lancets in a plastic container, such as an empty detergent bottle. Seal the container when it is about three-quarters full. Lancets are considered medical waste, so you'll want to check with your local trash collection agency about proper disposal.

URINE TESTING

If for some reason, you cannot perform SMBG, your doctor may advise that you test your urine for glucose using special test strips. However, this form of testing provides only a rough estimate of blood sugar levels and is far from ideal. This testing was more common years ago, but is not considered a good way to monitor blood sugar today. With the ease of use of glucose meters and the widespread availability, it is really hard to imagine that someone can't do some form of SMBG.

However, another form of urine testing, urine *ketone* testing, remains an important part of monitoring, especially if you have type 1 diabetes, gestational diabetes, or you are pregnant with preexisting diabetes. Ketones are a metabolic by-product of the fat-burning process created by a relative or absolute absence of insulin. Although ketones can be a source of cellular energy, they can be detrimental in large amounts and can cause a life-threatening emergency condition called ketoacidosis.

To test for ketones, dip a special test strip into your urine. In fifteen seconds to two minutes, the test strip changes color and you can then compare the strip to a color chart. If the result of urine ketone testing is positive, measures to increase hydration and increase insulin dosing may be needed. If the test is consistently positive, it is important to notify your provider.

If you have type 1 diabetes, you should test your urine for ketones when you are sick (have a cold, the flu, or other illness) or have nausea or vomiting; you are pregnant; or your blood glucose level is high (over 240 mg/dl). Your provider may want you to test under other conditions as well.

If you have type 2 diabetes, the chance of developing ketoacidosis is less. However, during severe illnesses, it is possible that ketoacidosis may develop in certain situations. It is therefore wise to test your urine for ketones when you get severely ill with a cold, flu, or other illness; you have nausea and vomiting; or your blood sugar is persistently high.

AT-HOME TESTING OF A1C

The self-monitoring you do at home provides an important snapshot of your blood sugar at the moment of testing. But as also stressed throughout this book, you'll also want to have your blood tested with an objective test, the A1c test, which measures average blood sugar levels over a three-month period and is the most accepted measure of overall diabetes control. A1c is the technical name for the test that measures the percent of glucose attached to hemoglobin, a protein in your red blood cells. Blood sugar binds to the hemoglobin and stays bound for the life of the cell, which is around three months. By measuring the amount of blood sugar attached to your hemoglobin, your doctor can get a very good reading of your average blood sugar levels for the past three months.

A1c is measured in percentages. People without diabetes have a level generally less than 6 percent, depending on the assay used. Unfortunately, average levels for Americans with diabetes are much higher, and have been suggested to be well above 7 percent as an average. This increased level is associated with a greater risk for complications. We now recommend people with diabetes keep levels below 7 percent at a minimum, and many suggest that we strive to normalize the A1c if it can be done without a lot of side effects. Small changes in A1c levels can make a big difference. Lowering levels just one point can reduce complications by 30 to 35 percent.

In the past, the only way to check your A1c was at the doctor's office — which is a good idea for accuracy. But you can also track your A1c levels at home. A company called Metrika makes a disposable, pager-sized A1c monitor called the A1cNow that you can buy for around twenty-five dollars at most major drugstores. This device gives your A1c reading in just five minutes from a small drop of blood. No prescription is required, and you don't have to wait for lab results. But, as you do with the SMBG, this home test should also agree with the A1c done at your doctor's office and be analyzed at a certified medical laboratory.

TAKING CHARGE

Clearly, daily blood sugar testing is a vital part of your regimen to manage diabetes. The appropriate schedule of testing that is right for you depends on your individual case. If you are on insulin injections, and take three to four injections a day, it will be imperative that you monitor more frequently to adjust your insulin as required. However, if you are following a good diet, and don't take medication on a daily basis, obviously, your frequency for home blood glucose checks will be less. It is best to discuss an appropriate schedule with your diabetes health-care team.

You are in control of your diabetes; it is not in control of you. Every time you check your blood sugar, every time you follow your diet, every time you make a healthy choice—you outwit and take charge of this disease. A normal, healthy life is not only possible, but probable. Self-monitoring of your blood sugar is another tool you should use to make that promise a reality.

SPECIAL CONDITIONS: TESTING IF YOU'RE ILL

If you become ill or stressed, your blood sugar can rise. Under either of these conditions, you'll want to take some extra measures. For example:

• Test your blood glucose more frequently and record the results.

• Contact your provider about possibly adjusting your medication if you are unable to eat, especially in the presence of ketones.

• Drink plenty of fluids.

• Test your urine for ketones during times of illness (e.g., vomiting, diarrhea, etc.), especially if you are an individual with type 1 diabetes.

• Contact your doctor immediately if any of the following occur: your blood sugar stays 300 mg/dl or higher; ketonuria (ketones in your urine); vomiting or diarrhea, mental clouding; trouble breathing; or evidence of infection.

*

9

$$\Big[\;\text{Keeping the Momentum:}\;\Big]$$

Keeping the Momentum: Reap the Benefits of Outside Support

WHENEVER I HAVE A PATIENT IN MY office with a new diagnosis of diabetes, I can see the fear and uncertainty on his or her face. I tell my patients that there are two important things to remember. First, there is something they can do about it, and second, this is a disease with which they can live a perfectly normal life. This is challenging, because most people aren't emotionally ready for what's ahead. You know yourself that one of the hardest parts of dealing with diabetes is the toll the disease takes on you mentally. Many people either deny they have it or get angry or depressed about it. But while such reactions may be normal, they can be harmful if you don't work through them and then refocus your energy into taking care of yourself. If you've been recently diagnosed, it is natural to want to deny that you have it. But you must get past that point. There is a way to do this, and it comes in the form of health-care professionals and other people with diabetes. Outside support like this enables you to cope and learn, to help while being helped, and to find hope. It can make a real, measurable difference in your life.

The more you know about your body, and the more you understand diabetes, the better your chances that you can effectively manage diabetes and prevent the progression of complications. When you have a real grasp of why diet, exercise, and medication must be part of your life, it is so much easier for you to stay on the road you must now travel for the rest of your life. Whether you have prediabetes, type 1 diabetes, or type 2 diabetes, you are not alone, and the millions of people who share your plight—and those who coordinate their care—are a tremendous resource that you need and can help you keep on track with your program. Just remember, "No man is an island."

The results of the Diabetes Prevention Program (DPP) showed that ongoing education and support significantly reduced the risk of developing diabetes in people of all ages. You can tap into those resources very easily by taking advantage of diabetes educational programs that offer an interdisciplinary team approach. This involves you, your provider, diabetes educators, a dietitian, pharmacist, an exercise specialist, and others. With the help of your team, you learn about nutrition management, exercise therapy, medication management, monitoring your blood sugar, and how to cope with many of the emotional issues relating to diabetes. Certainly, diabetes can have a dramatic effect on your life, but it doesn't have to be debilitating. With a support team and access to the right information, you can take charge of your life. Here is a closer look at how to put together your own support team:

A Prescription for Building a Support Team

You

The latest approach to diabetes management puts you in charge. After all, diabetes affects many aspects of your life. And because nobody knows your life better than you do, you must step into the role of the quarterback of your diabetes-care team in order to get your treatment needs met. As quarterback, you choose the professionals who best serve your needs, help you track your progress, and keep you focused on your goals.

You'll want to surround yourself with knowledgeable, trustworthy, expert people who can help you get the information, advice, treatments, and support you need to manage your diabetes effectively. The support people you'll need are described in the sections below. As you go about putting your team together, remember that these people work for you. You have enlisted them to help you learn about diabetes, understand how it specifically affects you, and provide you with the tools, education, and resources that empower you to make your own informed health-care decisions.

Your Physician

You'll want to be under the care of a doctor who not only has skill and training in treating diabetes, but also who will support and work with you. Together, you and your provider should develop a good working relationship where there is mutual understanding, respect, listening, and trust. You should feel comfortable talking with and asking questions of your doctor. This is so important to your ongoing care and health.

One way to find the right doctor is to contact the American Diabetes Association (ADA) (www.diabetes.org or 800-DIABETES). This organization can provide you with a list of the doctors who specialize in diabetes. Another avenue is to call your local medical society and ask for a list of doctors who care for patients with diabetes. These physicians will include those who are board certified in endocrinology (the specialty that focuses on hormonal disorders, such as diabetes), or who specialize in internal medicine or family medicine and are board certified in those specialties. "Board certification" means your doctor has met the most rigorous training and continuing education offered in his or her field of medicine. It is important to note that there are simply not enough endocrinologists in the United States to care for all the individuals with diabetes, and the majority of diabetes care is indeed delivered by internists and family medicine specialists. It is also important to note that family nurse practitioners or physician's assistants who work with your doctor can be an integral part of your care. The important thing is to find a provider with whom you can communicate, who is willing to work for you. Your diabetes condition may ultimately require a specialist, and your primary-care provider can refer you to a specialist when you need one.

Your Diabetes Educator

After you find a doctor, add a diabetes educator to your team. To be honest, these individuals are most often a patient's best advocate and the person you will confide in most often. Diabetes educators, in my opinion, are *the* most vital part of any diabetes support team. Most often, a diabetes educator will also be a nurse, dietitian, or pharmacist by training. If possible, choose a certified diabetes educator (CDE), a trained health professional who is certified by the National Certification Board for Diabetes Educators to teach people with diabetes how to manage the disease. CDEs must have at least two years and one thousand hours of experience in diabetes education, be currently employed as a diabetes educator, and have successfully completed a comprehensive examination covering diabetes. As with your doctor, you should feel comfortable with your educator and free to ask questions about the practical details of diabetes care.

Specifically, your diabetes educator provides information and one-on-one guidance on managing diabetes, and instruction on blood sugar monitoring. He or she should also address issues relating to high and low blood sugars, care during illness, preventing long-term complications, foot care, and psychological aspects of diabetes. Your diabetes educator can help motivate you to plan behavior changes to maintain the best control of your disease. An educator also teaches classes on diabetes management and shares resources available on local, state, and national levels. Your provider or health plan may be able to refer you to a certified diabetes educator, or you can contact the American Association of Diabetes Educators (AADE) (www.aadenet.org) for the names of diabetes educators in your area.

Registered Dietitian

It is a good idea to have a dietitian on your team. This professional can help you plan your diet, teach you how foods affect blood sugar, determine food portions, show you how to read labels, give advice on eating out choices and healthy cooking techniques, and instruct you in how to adjust your meal plans to activities and illness. Some dietitians are also certified diabetes educators. A "registered" dietitian is someone who has passed a national examination sponsored by the Commission on Dietetic Registration (CDR). To find a registered dietitian who specializes in diabetes in your area, go to the

Web site of the American Dietetic Association (www.eatright.org) and follow the link called Find a Nutrition Professional.

Exercise Physiologist or Physical Therapist

Exercise is important because it helps you feel better physically and manage the stress of dealing with diabetes more effectively. There are two types of exercise specialists who can aid a diabetes patient: an exercise physiologist, someone who has a university degree in exercise science; or a physical therapist, a specialist trained to work with patients to restore their activity, strength, and motion following an illness or injury. Either of these specialists can help you understand how exercise impacts the management of your diabetes. They have special training to help you develop exercise plans that can make you healthier, and they can assist you in designing a plan to help you lose weight and become more fit. Because blood glucose levels are an issue with exercise, these professionals can show you how to balance food and diabetes medication to keep diabetes from interfering with regular exercising. Unfortunately, in the majority of cases, the diabetes team you put together may not have the support of these individuals because of availability in the local area or resources to support their involvement. But, if they are part of your team, they are very valuable to your overall program.

Another option may be a personal trainer who guides you through strength training and/or aerobic workouts. Personal trainer certification is another critical element in finding a knowledgeable trainer. Locate a trainer who is certified, but also realize that the majority of personal trainers may not have the underlying knowledge of the diabetes disease state. So, they may not be as helpful in answering questions regarding medication use combined with the exercise program. It would be important to work with your provider in this regard and to definitely let them know about the exercise program.

Pharmacist

A pharmacist can help you manage your medications, if you have to take oral diabetes drugs or use insulin. He or she can review how these medications work in the body, how they are dosed, and what side effects you might expect. Additionally, your pharmacist is an excellent source of information about possible interactions with other medications as well as how medications that aren't taken for diabetes may affect your blood sugar. Today, given all the medications that are available and the fact that interactions may occur, the pharmacist is an invaluable resource to your diabetes program.

Mental Health Counselor

Feeling sad or down, or stressed from coping with the disease? These are common, understandable reactions to having diabetes. When that blue feeling or strain lasts more than a few weeks or really begins to interfere with your daily life or with taking care of your diabetes, you may be suffering from depression or anxiety. Both are biochemical conditions, and not a defect in your character. They can be treated with therapy or medications, and both will improve your mood and functioning. Your physician may elect to treat this condition himself after discussing this issue with you. Alternatively, he or she may feel you could benefit by being referred to a mental health counselor—a psychologist, psychiatrist, or social worker—who can guide you in terms of thinking more positively and productively about yourself and your life. If you need a specialist, choose a therapist who has experience in counseling people with diabetes. You may want to consult a psychiatrist; he or she can prescribe antidepressants if needed. Of course, if you suspect that you may be suffering from depression, you should discuss this with your doctor.

Diabetes Education Programs

Most hospitals and medical centers offer a series of weekly classes where you can learn about practically every aspect of diabetes management, from basic information to advanced level skills, in a small supportive group. You can take your partner, family, or other support person to attend with you. Class time is often divided among a diabetes educator, a dietitian, nurse, exercise physiologist, physicians, and other medical experts. These classes provide an invaluable learning opportunity, advanced information, and skills that will help you immeasurably in managing a healthy lifestyle. Call your hospital or talk to your provider about the availability of diabetes classes.

Self-Help Groups

Coping with diabetes can be challenging, but support groups can make it easier. Such groups offer psychological support and help educate you on leading healthful lifestyles, including proper nutrition, exercise, and the importance of getting regular care. You can also learn about complications associated with diabetes, such as stroke, blindness, or kidney failure. Most important, support groups give you the opportunity to talk to other people with diabetes who can understand you because they are in a similar situation. The support you get provides not only information and new ideas, but also empathy. You listen to one another, then affirm and validate what each member of the group has to say and contribute. In a good support group, you'll have the freedom to talk and experience an understanding and acceptance that can be hard to find anywhere else.

After Sarah, age fifty-four, was diagnosed with type 2 diabetes, she felt confused—and alone. She knew what problems diabetes could cause the body—heart disease, kidney problems, blindness, and other complications— but she didn't know what could be done to avert them. "I felt powerless," she said. "I had gone through most of my life feeling like I had some control over events. But the diagnosis of diabetes, well, that control seemed to vanish. How could I regain control of my body?"

Sarah was put in contact with a diabetes support group affiliated with a local hospital, and she began to attend weekly meetings. What Sarah found was a gathering of people who were just like her—they had been diagnosed with diabetes and were all learning how to manage it successfully. "Everyone was in the same boat," she recalled. "Many of us had experienced similar feelings about the disease. I felt relieved, really, that there were people with diabetes, just like me, who had managed to control it and not have it control their lives."

True, Sarah had to face the brutal truth of her diabetes, but it was empowering for her to learn that, yes, she could deal with issues over which she had control. "From being involved in my diabetes support group, I learned that how we handle our illness is a choice. Sure, we can whine and complain and get depressed, or we can choose to do something about it. Now when I get up in the morning, I tell myself that I, not my diabetes, have the power to guide my life. That's one of the many lessons I learned from my support group. It gave me hope, and it made me feel in control again."

More people with diabetes should take advantage of support groups. These groups are where you find the motivation you need. A support group gives you and your family a feeling of hope. You get to know people in your group like family, and you draw strength and support from them. This is really a wonderful thing. Ask your provider or diabetes educator, or call 1-800-DIABETES or your local hospital, to find out about diabetes support groups in your area.

Internet Support

Many Web-based health management services have popped up on the Internet to help better manage your diabetes, particularly your blood sugar control. These services have features such as self-management tools and automatic uploads of blood sugar levels from glucometers. With other easy-to-use-tools, you can plan, track, and report related data, such as food intake, exercise, and vital signs, and share a complete health profile with their health-care providers via the Internet. Be very careful with this approach, however. If you choose to do this, it is highly recommended that you share the details of this service with your physician or certified diabetes educator. You should provide the specific recommendations to be offered from the Internet and have them reviewed by your doctor or certified nurse educator. You want to be certain that the program offered is indeed one that is in line with your requirements and offers advice based on sound medical experience and research.

Many of these sites offer customized meal and fitness plans to eliminate guesswork. You can use dietitian-designed meal systems, create your own plans, or access menus from national chain restaurants, all complete with full caloric and nutritional values. Some have live chat features, as well as ongoing feedback on your progress.

In a twelve-month study published in *Diabetes Care,* 104 patients with diabetes and A1c of 9 or higher completed a diabetes education class and were randomized to continue with their usual care or receive Web-based care management. The latter group received a notebook computer, glucose and blood pressure monitoring devices, and access to a care management Web site. The Web site provided educational modules, accepted uploads from monitoring devices, and had an internal messaging system for patients to communicate with their care manager. By the end of the experimental period, people receiving Web-based care management had a lower A1c when compared with the other group. Interestingly, those who used the Web site most faithfully had the lowest A1c numbers. Additionally, people with high blood pressure in the Web-based group had the greatest reductions in blood pressure. Also impressive, HDL cholesterol rose and triglycerides fell in the

Web-based group. These findings led the researchers to conclude: "Web-based care management may be a useful adjunct in the care of patients with poorly controlled diabetes."

Clearly, Internet support, especially in today's world, has the potential to be a valid and effective way to manage diabetes. It really helps to have other people encouraging you, and this resource is another way to get that level of support. However, as stated previously, before embarking on any program on the Internet, it is important that your health-care team be advised of the program and the program content to make sure it is based on sound medical advice. Because there are so many sites on the Internet, here are some suggestions for picking the best one(s) for you:

- Don't rely on just one site; look at a variety—because no matter how objective a site is or seems to be, there are still biases. For example, a number of Web sites are sponsored by companies that have particular products, such as medications, to promote. Again, have the specifics of the site reviewed by your physician or diabetes educator.
- For solid mainstream diabetes advice, look to Web sites run by government agencies, state health departments, universities, hospitals, and medical centers. (I've listed several of these in the Appendix C.)
- If you need support but without going to an actual support group, try chat rooms, bulletin boards, and an online support group.

Other Important Team Members

You won't need every specialist or professional I've mentioned on your team; your choices depend on the state and progression of your diabetes. In addition, your team will also depend on the availability of these individuals in your local area. In addition to the individuals mentioned earlier, other medical practitioners will be important in your care; these may include the following:

Ophthalmologist. This is a physician who specializes in the medical and surgical care of the eyes and visual system and in the prevention of eye disease and injury. Ophthalmologists provide a full range of care that includes routine eye exams, diagnosis and medical treatment of eye disorders and diseases, prescriptions for eyeglasses, surgery, and management of eye problems that are caused by illnesses and diseases. Ophthalmologists can be medical doctors (M.D.) or doctors of osteopathy (D.O.). If you have eye problems related to diabetes, it is best to consult with an ophthalmologist who specializes in diabetic eye disease.

Podiatrist. A podiatric physician deals with the diagnosis, treatment, and prevention of diseases of the human foot. Among the disorders treated include bunions, heel pain/spurs, hammertoes, neuromas, ingrown toenails, warts, corns, and calluses. The podiatric physician treats sprains, fractures, infections, and injuries of the foot, ankle, and heel. Find a podiatrist who is experienced in diabetes-related foot problems.

Cardiologist. A cardiologist is a doctor who specializes in diagnosing, treating, and preventing diseases or conditions of the cardiovascular system, which includes the heart and blood vessels. Cardiology is a subspecialty of internal medicine.

Nephrologist. This specialist is a physician who has been educated and trained in kidney diseases, kidney transplantation, and dialysis therapy. Nephrologists treat many different kidney disorders, electrolyte disorders, kidney stones, high blood pressure, acute kidney disease, and end-stage renal disease. Nephrology is a subspecialty of internal medicine.

Working with Your Diabetes Care Team

I encourage you to take an active role in your treatment by preparing for your checkups and staying on top of your health. Each time you meet with your physician, be sure to take your blood sugar record with you (see page 223). You'll want to check it for trends and point these out to your doctor. Also, take an advocate, such as a family member or trusted friend, with you to your appointments, in case you feel anxious about your checkups and have trouble remembering everything that was discussed.

Keep a treatment log (see the example below). Its purpose is to keep track of the tests and treatments you've had, your appointments, contact information for each of your team members, and other important information. You'll want to keep a record of all prescription drugs and any nonprescription medicines, vitamins, minerals, and natural products you're taking—as well as the strength and dose of each. In some cases, you may be seeing more than one doctor, and it is important that each one knows what the other has prescribed for you and what over-the-counter products you take so that together you can avoid dangerous interactions. Not only is it important to know what you're taking, it is vital to know why you're taking it, and what side effects or warning signs may occur. It is, after all, your body, and you shouldn't put anything in it that you don't understand. Be sure to note in your treatment log any side effects or unusual symptoms you experience that you suspect may be connected to your medications. That way, you can ask about them the next time you talk to your doctor.

I also recommend you keep a running list of questions you have so that you can ask your team. Jot them down as they occur to you. Often, under the pressure of limited time or anxiety during your appointment, you can easily forget questions that otherwise seemed so clear just the day prior. Also, prioritize your questions so the most important questions are answered first.

Whenever you have an appointment or session with one of your team members, take time to prepare. Be sure to bring your treatment log, as well as your blood glucose information and meter, and any other information that pertains to the support person with whom you're meeting. Remember, you are the one in charge of your care. That goal—taking care of your diabetes and yourself—is absolutely vital to your quality of life.

My Treatment Log
My Diabetes Care Team

Name	Specialty	Office Number	Mobile Number

(continued)

My Treatment Log
(continued)

Medications I'm Taking

Medication	Dose	When to Take It

Nutritional Supplements/Over-the-Counter Medicines I'm Taking

Medication	Dose	When to Take It

My blood sugar targets are: _____ to _____ before meals to _____ after meals

Blood pressure target: _____ / _____ or less

My weight target: _____ pounds

My current weight is: _____ pounds

Last A1c test result: _____ percent (date tested: _____)

(This test tells you if your blood glucose has been under control for the past three months; A1c test result should be less than 7 percent.)

My next A1c test due on: _____

My next physical exam: _____

Discuss the Following with My Health-Care Team

- A1c, blood pressure
- Cholesterol (LDL)
- Other test results

(continued)

My Treatment Log
(continued)

- Meal plan
- Nutritional supplements
- Exercise plan
- Medications/side effects
- Glucose self-monitoring plan
- Foot care
- New or unusual symptoms
- Other questions I have

My Upcoming Appointments

Appointment	Date	Time

Part 3

Medical Management

Optimizing Your Antidiabetes Medications

I'M SURE YOU'D LIKE TO EAT HEALTHY and get more active—two of the cornerstones of treatment for type 2 diabetes—to control your blood sugar and not have to fool with medication, and certainly not with insulin. But the reality is, you may have to take medication—and that is a good thing, because we know from research that it has a powerful effect on helping you stay healthy.

If you've faithfully followed your diet and exercise program, and have even lost weight, yet your blood sugar is not within the target range suggested by your health-care team, then you will most likely be prescribed an oral antidiabetes drug or insulin. Having to take antidiabetes medicine doesn't mean you've failed, but based on the natural history of the process, it is to be expected. As we discussed, over time, the ability of your pancreas to produce insulin may diminish. So, it simply means you will need medications to help with any underlying problems that have progressed due to diabetes.

The benefits of drug therapy have been shown conclusively in large clinical trials, particularly the largest study of type 2 diabetics ever conducted: the United Kingdom Prospective Diabetes Study, which I've described elsewhere in this book. In this study, which involved more than five thousand patients, improved blood sugar control emerged unequivocally as the key to preventing and controlling complications from the disease.

Because diabetic complications progress over decades—and are largely silent before the most serious damage occurs—this study was the first true look at what produces the best outcomes in long-term diabetes management. The results were conclusive: maintaining blood sugar control is critical for all people with diabetes from the onset of the disease. The key to absolute maintenance of that control is through drug therapy, whether with oral drugs or insulin, combined with your lifestyle changes. The study also found that the progression of microvascular complications of diabetes can be slowed down with tighter blood sugar control through oral therapy as well as with insulin.

There are many different oral antidiabetes drugs, and they work to control your blood glucose in different ways. Some boost your insulin in your bloodstream in response to an increase in your blood sugar. Others increase the sensitivity of your body to insulin. Still others work directly on your liver, blocking its production of glucose and thereby reducing levels of sugar in your bloodstream. Even if your diabetes has progressed, several of these drugs can be used together to get the best outcome for you as it relates to blood sugar control.

If you are like many people with type 2 diabetes, you may not be reaping the full benefits of your current antidiabetes drug program nor may you be aware of the latest additions to the antidiabetes drug arsenal. In this chapter, I'll help you make the most of those medications by reviewing the various oral agents that are available.

Traditional Medications for Type 2 Diabetes

Managing diabetes and lowering your blood sugar are challenging, but there is no need to ever feel discouraged. You can do it, and medications can help you. Most people with type 2 diabetes take medicine to help control their blood sugar levels, and many take more than one medicine to help treat diabetes in different ways. There are now five major classes of oral medications used to treat type 2 diabetes, and these are explained below. Your doctor will work with you to decide which one(s) are best for you.

Secretagogues

SULFONYLUREAS *(SUL-fah-nil-YOO-ree-ahs)* AND MEGLITINIDES *(meh-GLIT-in-ides)*

Secretagogues (*si-KREE-tuh-gawgs*) increase the secretion of your body's own insulin. Specifically, they work on the beta cells in the pancreas (the cells that produce the insulin) to stimulate greater production of insulin, thus lowering your blood sugar. Should type 2 diabetes worsen, as it may do, beta cells lose their function, so over time, these drugs may lose their effectiveness, and you may be switched to another form of drug therapy.

There are two subclasses of secretagogues: *sulfonylureas* and *meglitinides*. Sulfonylureas have been on the market for many years, as they were one of the first classes available for treatment of type 2 diabetes. They are divided into whether they are first generation (older meds), which include Diabinese (chlorpropamide) and Orinase (tolbutamide).

The second generation sulfonylureas (newer agents) include: Amaryl (glimepiride); Glucotrol and Glucotrol XL (glipizide); DiaBeta, Glynase, and Micronase (glyburide). Generally, if you are prescribed a sulfonylurea, it will most likely be a second generation drug.

The two meglitinides approved for use are Prandin (repaglinide) and Starlix (nateglinide). Sulfonylureas and secretagogues do a commendable job of helping improve glucose levels and, on average, reduce A1c levels by approximately 1 percent.

How to Take Them: Sulfonylureas may be given or prescribed once or twice daily, depending on the specific drug. Your doctor will tell you how many times a day you should take your diabetes pill(s). The time you take your pill depends on which specific drug you are prescribed. If you take your pill once a day, you will likely take it just before the first meal of the day (breakfast). If you take the medicine twice a day, you will likely take your first pill just before your first meal, and the second pill just before the last meal of the day (dinner). Take the medicine at the same times each day.

As for the meglitinides, Prandin is taken from thirty minutes before to just before a meal. It has an effect for the first few hours after the meal. Starlix is taken three times daily, with each major meal.

Side Effects: The most common side effects of sulfonylureas include a low blood sugar reaction (hypoglycemia) and weight gain. More infrequent complaints are an upset stomach, a skin rash, or itching. Hypoglycemia is a side effect of Prandin and Starlix.

Sulfonylureas

Drug	Dosages	Dosing Interval
Amaryl (glimepiride)	Starting dose = 1 or 2 mg, Maximum is 8 mg	Once daily
Diabinese (Chlorpropamide)	100 mg to 250 mg	Once daily
Glucotrol and Glucotrol XL (glipizide)	Starting dose = 5 mg Maximum recommended dose = 40 mg, but generally maximum effect is approximately 10 mg	Once daily or in divided doses
Diabeta, Glynase, and Micronase (glyburide)	Starting dose = 2.5–5 mg Maximum recommended dose = 20 mg, but generally maximum effect at approx. 10 mg or less	Once daily or in divided doses
Orinase	Starting dose = 1000 to 2000 mg Maximum recommended dose = 3000 mg	In divided doses, one before the morning meal, the other before the evening meal

Meglitinides

Drug	Dosages	Dosing Interval
Prandin (repaglinide)	Starting dose may be 0.5 mg to 1–2 mg, depending on your initial blood glucose and whether you have been treated previously. Maximum daily dosage = 16 mg	Most effective if taken at the start of a meal, 15 or 30 minutes before the meal
Starlix (nateglinide)	Starting dose = 60–120 mg with each meal Maximum recommended dose = 120 mg three times daily	Three times a day, with each major meal

Biguanides *(by-GWAN-ides)*

Glucophage (metformin) is the only biguanide approved for use in the United States. It lowers blood sugar by making sure your liver does not produce too much sugar. Metformin may also help your tissues become more efficient when using insulin. You may lose some weight when you start to take metformin. Metformin can also improve blood fat and cholesterol levels, which are often abnormal if you have type 2 diabetes. Metformin has been shown in studies to reduce A1c by 1 to 2 percent. It is now one of the most common medications for type 2 diabetes and, in the majority of cases, is the agent your doctor most likely will start first. Metformin is one of the medicines that proved effective in diabetes prevention studies and is now a mainstay for diabetes treatment worldwide.

How to Take It: Metformin is generally taken twice a day, usually with a morning or evening meal. The starting dose is 500 to 850 milligrams. The maximum recommended dosage is 2,500 milligrams.

Side Effects: Common side effects of metformin are diarrhea, nausea, vomiting, abdominal bloating, and gas. These generally improve the longer you are on the medication. Metformin can cause a rare but serious side effect called *lactic acidosis,* a buildup of lactic acid in your blood that can cause serious damage. Lactic acidosis is a medical emergency that must be treated in a hospital. It occurs mostly in people whose kidneys are not working normally. Although rare, lactic acidosis can be fatal in up to half the people who develop it. Some of the symptoms include feeling very weak, tired, or uncomfortable, unusual muscle pain, and rapid breathing that you can't explain. But, as stated, this is a very rare side effect. As such, based on how well it works, metformin remains as one of the more prescribed and effective medications used for type 2 diabetes today.

Alpha-Glucosidase Inhibitors *(al-fa-GLU-co-side-ase)*

These drugs work quite differently from other diabetes medications. They block enzymes that digest starches in the small intestines. This slows the digestion of carbohydrates, which, in turn, slows the rise in the blood sugar after you eat a meal. This slower rise in glucose level matches your reduced internal production of insulin to improve blood sugar control. You're not as likely to experience the elevations that may be seen in blood sugar after meals. The two medications in this class are Precose (acarbose) and Glyset (miglitol).

How to Take Them: Both drugs are usually taken three times a day with the first bite of each main meal. The starting dose is 25 milligrams before meals; the maximum recommended dose is 100 milligrams three times daily before meals.

Side Effects: Common side effects with Precose are abdominal pain, diarrhea, and gas. The side effects of Glyset are similar: gas, soft stools, diarrhea, or abdominal discomfort. These reactions subside with time, but unfortunately, these side effects have limited the use of these agents in the United States.

Thiazolidinediones *(THIGH-ah-ZO-li-deen-DYE-owns)*

Thiazolidinediones are a class of drugs that help your body use its own natural insulin better and thus decrease insulin resistance. This lowers your blood sugar. There are two thiazolidinediones on the market: Avandia (rosiglitazone) and Actos (pioglitazone). Studies show that thiazolidinediones can reduce A1c by 1 to 2 percent.

Avandia can be taken alone or with other diabetes medicines, since many people need to take more than one medicine to help treat diabetes in different ways. Avandia is also available in combination with other diabetes medicines: Avandamet, a combination of Avandia and metformin; and Avandaryl, a combination of Avandia and glimepiride.

Actos is available in two combinations: with the sulfonylurea glimepiride as Duetact; and in combination with metformin as Actoplus Met. Actos tar-

Thiazolidinediones

Drug	Dosages	Dosing Interval
Avandia (rosiglitazone)	Starting dose = 4 mg Maximum daily dose = 8 mg	Single dose once a day or in divided doses twice a day
Actos (pioglitazone)	Starting dose = 15 mg or 30 mg Maximum daily dose = 45 mg	Should be taken once a day without regard to meal times

gets insulin resistance, and metformin acts primarily by reducing the amount of glucose produced by the liver.

How to Take Them: Actos and Avandia may be taken once or twice daily, depending on the dosage.

As for combination therapies, Avandamet is taken twice a day, with meals; and Avandaryl, once a day with your first main meal. Duetact is also taken once a day with your first main meal; and Actoplus is given once a day or in divided doses, with meals.

With any of these medicines, your doctor may need to increase the dosage to better control your blood glucose. Do not change your dose unless told to do so by your doctor.

Side Effects: Common side effects of the thiazolidinediones are weight gain and fluid retention.

As outlined, thiazolidinediones have been shown to be effective glucose-lowering agents. However, recently the cardiovascular safety for certain agents of this class has been called into question. Specifically, these drugs have been promoted as medication that may reduce heart disease based on their effectiveness regarding certain risk factors. However, studies that evaluated endpoints such as heart attack and other cardiovascular factors seem to suggest an increased risk for heart disease with use of particular agents from this class. We do know that patients with underlying heart disease or with other chronic conditions may have a higher risk for heart disease, including developing congestive heart failure, a condition that has been associated with use of thiazolidinediones. Thus, a detailed discussion needs to occur with your physician to determine if you are an appropriate candidate for this class of agents.

The Newest Antidiabetes Drugs

Today we have a large arsenal of therapeutic options, and the development and introduction of new drugs for diabetes continues. The latest medications are discussed below. Keep in mind, however, that while these new diabetes drugs and technologies are wonderful, you, the patient, are the key. Being compliant with drug therapy and following your doctor's guidelines can make a huge difference in your health.

Januvia *(jah-NEW-vee-ah)* (sitagliptin) and Galvus *(GAL-vus)* (vildagliptin)

Januvia (currently available) and Galvus (FDA approval pending) are both from of a new class of oral drugs for type 2 diabetes called DPP-4 (dipeptidyl peptidase-IV) inhibitors. DPP-4 is an enzyme in your body that breaks down a protein called glucagon-like peptide 1 (GLP-1). GLP-1 is released after meals and helps to increase insulin secretion from your pancreas. GLP-1 has other effects, such as regulating the amount of sugar produced by your liver and regulating the rate by which the stomach empties. GLP-1 doesn't stay very long in your blood because it is broken down. Scientists realized that if they could stop DPP-4 from degrading the GLP-1 so rapidly, GLP-1 levels can rise after a meal, and therefore exert all the known effects known for this protein that regulate blood sugar levels.

How It Works: Galvus and Januvia increase your body's own natural supply of GLP-1, a naturally available hormone that is produced by the intestines after a meal, by preventing their breakdown. The DPP-4 inhibitors such as Galvus and Januvia block the enzyme DPP-4, which breaks down GLP-1. As a result of the increase in your body's own GLP-1, the pancreas produces more insulin and the liver makes less blood glucose. These drugs generally don't cause weight gain.

How to Take It: Galvus and Januvia can be taken orally once a day.

Side Effects: Hypoglycemia is less likely to occur with these agents when compared with other secretagogues. Generally, they are well tolerated, but side effects include cold and flulike symptoms and headaches.

Byetta (exenatide)

The launch of this interesting drug can be traced to a researcher's curiosity in the eating habits of the Gila monster, a lizard native to several southwestern U.S. states. The Gila monster can go for long periods without eating. In fact, it eats only four times a year. During the time it is not eating, its insulin-producing pancreas is not active. When the lizard finally does eat, a hormone (exentin) secreted in its saliva reactivates the pancreas. Exendin also affects the lizard's blood sugar through influences on the pancreas. Byetta (exenatide) is in many ways similar to exendin.

How It Works: Byetta works in four different ways. First, it signals your pancreas to release more insulin after you eat a meal. Second, it acts to reduce glucagon, a hormone in your body that works in the liver to promote high blood sugar after meals, thus keeping glucose normalized. Third, it delays the emptying of food from your stomach, which also helps prevent high glucose levels after you eat. Finally, in clinical trials, Byetta has been shown to help reduce the appetite and assist people in losing weight. It is not unusual to see significant weight loss for patients maintained on Byetta.

How to Take It: Byetta is an injectable administered by a pen-delivery system. The pen is prefilled with your daily doses of the medicine, so you do not have to worry about measuring each dose. Also, it works when used with other medication taken by mouth such as metformin, secretagogues, and, like Glucophage (*metformin*), thiazolidinediones to help keep your blood sugar under control.

Side Effects: The most common side effect with Byetta is mild-to-moderate nausea, which decreases over time in most people. If you have nausea, your health-care professional can give you tips on how to manage it. There is also an increased risk of developing hypoglycemia, particularly if you are taking a sulfonylurea with Byetta. In this case, your provider will most likely reduce your sulfonylurea dose to reduce the chance of low blood sugar.

Symlin *(SIM-lin)* (pramlintide acetate)

Symlin (pramlintide acetate) is another injectable medicine that helps to control blood sugar for adults with type 2 diabetes who are on insulin injections. It is also given to people with type 1 diabetes. Currently, it is only recommended to be used with mealtime insulin to control blood sugar. With Symlin, you may be able to reduce your blood sugar swings, lose weight, and use less of the fast-acting insulin before meals.

How It Works: Symlin is indicated if your blood sugar is noted to be consistently high after meals, despite being on a fast-acting insulin before meals. One reason erratic swings may occur is that your body may be missing or may not have enough of a hormone called amylin. Under normal conditions, amylin works with insulin to control how quickly sugar enters your blood from your stomach after meals. Without enough amylin, you may experience high blood sugar levels after meals. In the absence of amylin, insulin may be less effective in lowering these spikes, and consequently, your blood sugar may stay above normal and be hard to control.

Symlin works with your insulin to better control blood sugar levels after meals. Symlin also helps food move out of your stomach at a slower rate, which helps control the rate at which sugar enters the blood following meals. Further, it reduces the amount of sugar that the liver sends into the bloodstream after meals and helps regulate your food intake by decreasing appetite. One of the benefits of Symlin is its ability in many cases to promote weight loss.

How to Take It: Symlin is used only in combination with insulin to help lower blood sugar during the three hours after meals. So, if you're on medication for diabetes that you take by mouth only, this drug is not indicated for you at this time. The amount of Symlin you use depends on whether you have type 1 or type 2 diabetes. Your doctor will determine the appropriate starting and maintenance doses. You inject Symlin under the skin (subcutaneously) of your stomach area (abdomen) or upper leg (thigh) and at least two inches away from your insulin injection site. Make sure you do not mix Symlin with insulin in the same syringe; this can alter the activity of your insulin.

Side Effects: Common side effects include nausea, vomiting, abdominal pain, headache, fatigue, dizziness, and hypoglycemia.

Which Antidiabetes Drugs Can Be Taken Together?

Each type of medication has its own way of lowering blood sugar. If your doctor advises an antidiabetes medication, you'll usually be started on one drug to see how it works over the course of two to three months. Should that regimen still not give you tight glucose control after that time period, your doctor may prescribe a second drug that is added to the other one. This approach is called combination therapy and is often effective for achieving tighter control.

A case in point: when I diagnosed him with type 2 diabetes five years earlier, Jonathan, age sixty, was about thirty pounds overweight. I prescribed metformin (Glucophage) and increased the dose to 1,000 milligrams twice daily over the years. Also, I counseled him to increase his physical activity and follow a prudent diet of lean proteins, complex carbohydrates, and reduced fat. However, he had been unable to stick to any of these lifestyle recommendations with any consistency.

On laboratory examination, his fasting blood glucose was 187 mg/dl; and his A1c, 9.1 percent. A random urine sample revealed microalbuminuria, and his blood lipids were: total cholesterol, 231 mg/dl; LDL cholesterol, 126 mg/dl; HDL cholesterol, 35 mg/dl; and triglycerides, 335 mg/dl. These laboratory results confirmed that he had both poor control of glucose levels and unacceptable cholesterol levels. In addition, he now had microalbuminuria, indicating early damage to his kidneys. Clearly, his diabetes was inadequately controlled and becoming progressively worse.

Since his initial visit, I added a thiazolidinedione to his regimen, as well as a statin added to control his elevated LDL ("bad" cholesterol). Due to the protein in his urine, I also prescribed an ACE inhibitor. He was encouraged to continue to try to make lifestyle modifications, and he was referred to a certified diabetes educator for additional reinforcement and reevaluation of his nutritional plan. The diabetes educator urged him to enhance his physical activity and begin a walking program.

The combination therapy with two oral medications helped reduce his A1c by approximately 1 percent down to a value of 8 percent, which was a good response. However, he was still not at his goal (recommended <7 percent) many months later; therefore, I prescribed one injection at night of a long-acting insulin (glargine) in addition to his two oral antidiabetic medications. This combination of insulin and two oral agents worked well to lower his A1c to less than 7 percent. Further, his cholesterol profile improved with the initiation and increasing dosage of the statin. His LDL ("bad" cholesterol) level dropped to 85 mg/dl. With his current medication protocol, combined with better lifestyle adjustments, he has succeeded in maintaining much better control, and has a good chance of preventing or delaying further complications.

An important point in this case is that the underlying processes causing diabetes continue to progress over time. But, that doesn't mean you can't continue to control the condition. In this case, advancing to two medications taken by mouth worked to improve control. Adding a single injection of a longer-acting insulin along with the two oral agents worked extremely well. Simply put, advancing therapy when needed did the job well. In addition, today we have agents like Byetta (exenatide) and Januvia (sitagliptin) that could have been used in this case.

How Can You Tell If Your Diabetes Medicines Are Working?

Some people stay on a certain pill for years; others may have to be switched because sometimes a drug loses its effectiveness. So if one doesn't work for you, your doctor can try another. The best way to monitor the effectiveness of any particular drug is to make sure the long-term and objective test to monitor glucose control, namely your A1c level, is acceptable. It is recommended that this level be below 7 percent at a minimum. If this test is still abnormal months after you take an effective dose of the medication or combination of medications, you may need to have your therapy advanced further as described in the case above. The important thing that you need to know is that if one regimen is not working to reduce your blood glucose within a reasonable time, approximately three to four months, it is time to advance therapy. One of the biggest problems we have today in diabetes management is that patients stay on therapeutic regimens that are ineffective for years. If that's your case, your average blood glucose remains high and this increases your chance of developing complications.

Clearly, your blood sugar tests when checked at home should reflect better control and should agree with the A1c test obtained at your recent visit to your provider. But studies have shown that complications are reduced when A1c levels are lowered, and this test is the definitive one to determine if your therapy is working. So, your target for the A1c test as suggested by the American Diabetes Association should be less than 7 percent. It is generally felt that the lower the A1c test is to normal, generally 6 percent or so, the better. But please be advised that as you try to improve your blood glucose to these levels, the chance of developing hypoglycemia increases.

Treating Hypoglycemia

One of the side effects with many diabetes drugs is hypoglycemia, or low blood sugar. This typically occurs when your blood glucose levels drop below the normal range (for example, less than 60 mg/dl). However, your blood glucose does not have to be below a certain value to have the symptoms of hypoglycemia. If there is a rapid drop from higher levels, you may feel the symptoms at a higher level of glucose other than 60 mg/dl or so. There are different degrees of severity. In mild cases of hypoglycemia, you'll feel hungry, a little irritable, and perhaps weak. If you have any of these early symptoms you will need some form of carbohydrate. The symptoms can be overcome by eating a meal or snack. Always carry a quick source of sugar, such as candy mints, sugar, honey, or glucose tablets or gels (available in pharmacies). The prompt treatment of mild hypoglycemic symptoms can prevent severe hypoglycemic reactions and raise your blood glucose level higher to relieve symptoms.

With more severe hypoglycemia, symptoms include clouding of your mental status and confusion, trembling, sweating, and a very rapid pulse. If prolonged, unconsciousness or convulsions can appear; this constitutes a medical emergency and requires immediate treatment. Permanent damage to the brain or even death may result if treatment is delayed. In these more severe cases, other individuals may be required to assist you and inject a hormone called glucagon into your muscles to help you recover. This is why it is so important that family members and friends know what to do if there is a problem.

Glucagon Emergency Kits

Medication, taken either by mouth or injection, has the potential to cause hypoglycemia, which is why it's a good idea to have a glucagon emergency

---

ASK DR. CEFALU: WHAT SHOULD I DO IF I GET SICK?

Be sure to continue taking your diabetes pills or insulin if you are on diabetes medication. However, if you are on a particular drug that increases insulin, your doctor may adjust it or stop it if you can't eat. Your physician may even advise you to take more insulin during an illness. Here are other precautions to take:

- Monitor your blood glucose frequently, and keep track of the results.
- Drink extra (calorie-free) liquids, and try to eat as you normally would. If you can't, try to have soft foods and liquids containing the equivalent amount of carbohydrates that you usually consume.
- Check your temperature every morning and evening. A fever may be a sign of infection.
- Call your doctor if any of the following happen to you: You feel too sick to eat normally and are unable to keep down food. You're having severe diarrhea. You have unexplained weight loss. Your temperature is higher than 101 degrees Fahrenheit. You have more frequent hypoglycemic episodes, or your blood sugar remains persistently high. You're having trouble breathing, or you feel sleepy or can't think clearly.

✳

---

kit on hand. It is available by prescription. This kit provides the hormone called glucagon, which is needed in severe cases of hypoglycemia. It must be used if you become severely hypoglycemic and are unable to take sugar by mouth. In a case like this, you'll need someone to give you an injection of glucagon, which increases your blood sugar by releasing stored glucose from the liver. Along with insulin, glucagon is a hormone responsible for the control of sugar in the blood. Make sure your family, friends, and coworkers know where to find and how to use the injection kit. Teach them how to give you an injection before an emergency arises. They can practice by giving you your normal insulin shots. It is important that they do so because a person who has never given a shot probably will not be able to do it in an emergency. You should be given glucagon if you are unconscious, are having a seizure, or do not improve after ingesting sufficient carbohydrates.

How to Avoid Drug Interactions

As part of controlling your diabetes and improving your health, you may be taking multiple medications—including high blood pressure drugs, cholesterol-lowering agents, painkillers—in addition to your diabetes drugs. These drugs can often interact with each other in untoward ways. Make sure your doctor is aware of any medications you now use, even if they are dietary supplements or over-the-counter preparations like aspirin or acetaminophen. There can be interactions between supplements and specific medicines, so if you are taking either, check with your doctor. In addition, one of the most valuable sources would be your pharmacist, who can provide information on possible interactions. In most cases, he or she will provide you with written information about the drug you are taking and also written information about interactions with other medications you take. Most pharmacies will also ask if you want to be counseled about the drug you are taking, and at that time, you may want to let them know about other medications you are on to determine if there will be a problem. Also, keep a list of all these medications, and tell your doctor about any side effect or reaction, even if it seems trivial.

Using Insulin: Not the Pain
It Used to Be

INTRODUCED IN THE 1920S, INSULIN IS A
life-saving treatment for many people with diabetes. If you have type 1 diabetes, your pancreas is severely damaged and you must use insulin in order
to survive. The vast majority of people with type 2 diabetes may eventually require insulin, given the natural history of the disease. So, if your doctor suggests you advance to insulin therapy, he or she is not punishing you. It simply
means you're at a stage in diabetes where your requirements for insulin are
greater than your body can produce. You are simply providing a hormone
that your body no longer produces in adequate amounts.

Of course, the drawback to insulin is that it must be injected, and many
people put off treatment with insulin because they don't like the thought
of injecting themselves. As a result, scientists have been on a quest to find
new insulin delivery technologies that do not require injection, and I will discuss those later in this chapter. Don't get me wrong. Injecting insulin is very
effective. In fact, I feel that more people with type 2 diabetes should use it,

in addition to making proper nutrition and lifestyle changes, earlier in the course of their disease if their blood sugar is not controlled. It's risky to delay advancing to insulin if your condition merits it. Insulin is not a last resort. If doctor puts you on insulin early, you can better control your blood sugar and reduce your risk of diabetes complications.

For decades, most insulin formulations were made from beef or pork pancreas or a combination of both. In the 1980s, manufacturers started using genetic engineering to modify insulin's amino acid sequence and produce versions that mimic the action of insulin made in the human pancreas. Since then, the Food and Drug Administration (FDA) has approved various "human" insulins, which are absorbed faster and cause fewer allergic reactions. There are now many forms of insulin available, and they are classified by how fast they start to work and how long their effects last. The types of insulin include rapid-acting, short-acting, intermediate-acting, and long-acting. Different types of insulin can be injected separately or mixed in the same syringe, and many rapid-acting insulins are premixed in the same syringe with a longer-acting insulin.

What Type of Insulin Is Best for You?

Whether you have type 1 or type 2 diabetes, insulin use must be balanced with diet and exercise. Your doctor will work with you to prescribe the type of insulin that is best for you. Deciding what type of insulin might be best for you, and how much, depends on many factors, including:

- Your body weight, activity level, food intake, and glucose control.
- Your willingness to give yourself multiple injections of insulin each day.
- How frequently you monitor your blood sugar level.

The following chart lists the types of injectable insulins with details about *onset* (the approximate time it takes insulin to reach your bloodstream and start reducing your blood glucose levels), *peak* (the period during which insulin is at its highest strength in terms of reducing blood glucose levels), and *duration* (how long insulin continues to work to lower blood glucose levels). The times provided in the table for the three factors are approximate times, and obviously may vary from patient to patient, depending on how you respond.

Type of Insulin (Brand Name)	Onset	Peak	Duration	When to Take This Insulin
Rapid-Acting				
Lispro (Humalog)	15–30 minutes	60 minutes	4–5 hours	Administer about 10 minutes before mealtime.
Aspart (NovoLog)	15–30 minutes	60 minutes	4–5 hours	Administer about 10 minutes before mealtime.
Glulisine (Apidra)	15–30 minutes	60 minutes	4–5 hours	Administer about 10 minutes before mealtime.
Short-Acting				
Regular (Humulin, Novolin)	30–60 minutes	2–4 hours	6–8 hours	Administer 30 to 60 minutes before a meal.
Intermediate-Acting				
NPH (Humulin N, Novolin N)	2–4 hours	4–6 hours	12–16 hours	Administer up to 1 hour prior to a meal.
Lente (Humulin L, Novolin L)	2–4 hours	4–12 hours	12–18 hours	Administer up to 1 hour prior to a meal.
Long-Acting				
Glargine (Lantus)	2 hours	No peak time; insulin is delivered at a steady level.	Approx. 24 hours	Administer once a day, at the same time each day.
Detemir (Levemir)	2 hours	May have peak effect	14–16 hours	Administer once or twice a day, irrespective of mealtime.

Premixed insulins are a combination of intermediate and short-acting or fast-acting insulins. Combinations such as 70/30 (70 intermediate/30 percent regular) and 75/25 (75 percent intermediate/25 percent fast-acting) are available in addition to other mixtures such as 50/50. As such, these premixed insulins will have the characteristics of combining the short- or fast-acting insulin and the properties of the intermediate-acting insulin.

Advanced Insulin Delivery Systems

If part of your treatment requires insulin injections, don't be upset. Millions of people take injections every day without thinking much about it. Over time, they've gotten used to the shots, and they come to appreciate the fact that insulin is making them feel better. I recommend that you talk to other people who use insulin. They'll tell you that the needles are so small and fine that they can barely be felt when puncturing the skin, and there is little pain or inconvenience. So rather than dwell on the injections, think of insulin as giving you the control you need to do what you want.

It is important to understand the normal function of the pancreas so as to understand why you take specific types of insulin. If you are nondiabetic, your pancreas produces insulin twenty-four hours a day at a low rate. This type of secretion is called "basal" insulin. It helps control your blood sugar between meals and maintain other processes important for your metabolism. You generally don't develop low blood sugar because you are also producing glucose (from your liver) in between meals.

When you eat a meal, you need to release increased amounts of insulin, called "bolus" or "prandial" (meaning "meal-related") insulin, to control the glucose that you ingested. At this stage, since you're taking in glucose orally, your liver should no longer make glucose. After the meal is digested in several hours, your insulin level declines to basal levels and your liver now starts releasing glucose again until your next meal. With this background, you now understand why you need both long-acting insulins to serve as basal insulin and regular and fast-acting insulins to serve as bolus or prandial insulin.

There are many ways to get insulin into the body, and most minimize pain. The majority of fast-acting and short-acting insulins available today can be given by insulin pens or by external insulin pumps. Here is a closer look at how these delivery systems work:

Syringe. Today's syringes are smaller and have finer needles that work to make injecting as easy and painless as possible. When insulin injections are done properly, you'll discover that this is relatively painless. Basically, a syringe system consists of a needle, barrel, and plunger. Your diabetes educator can teach you how to use the syringe, including proper disposal.

Insulin Pen. This device resembles an old-fashioned cartridge pen, only instead of a writing point, there's a needle, and instead of an ink cartridge, there's an insulin cartridge. Some pens are disposable, too. Insulin pens are convenient (especially if you travel and are on the go), accurate, and easy to use, particularly if you take at least three doses of insulin daily. Today, insulin pens are available for most of the insulin formulations and you simply can turn a dial to select the dose you need. Simply press a plunger to deliver the insulin.

External Insulin Pump. Insulin pump therapy delivers insulin in patterns similar to the way the human body delivers insulin. This gives you the flexibility to lead a more active, normal life. The pump is thus a good alternative to multiple daily injections for achieving glucose control. It attaches to your body through flexible tubing (catheter) and a needle inserted under your skin near your abdomen. In the newer products, the needle can be removed and only the catheter remains in place. A refillable cartridge holds enough insulin for several days, and you'll need to change needles and tubing at the recommended times. Insulin pumps are computerized devices, about the size of a deck of cards, and can be worn on your belt or in your pocket.

The pump delivers insulin in two ways: in a steady, measured, and continuous dose (the basal insulin) and as a surge (bolus) dose, at your direction, around mealtime. Certain factors may change the basal dose you require, however. These include exercise, illness, and medications. If you find you have gained weight or lost weight, this will most likely either increase or decrease, respectively, the basal insulin you need. Your doctor and health-care team can help you determine and set the appropriate adjustments.

To use a pump, however, you must check your blood glucose frequently and learn how to adjust insulin, food, and physical activity in response to those test results. You'll want to check with your insurance carrier before you buy a pump and all the supplies to see exactly what the cost will be to you, especially for the supplies after you have the pump in place. (Medicare may cover pumps and supplies for people with diabetes who meet certain eligibility requirements.)

This delivery system is popular with many patients, and they find it convenient. Robert, forty-nine, was diagnosed with type 2 diabetes several years ago. When oral medication failed to control his blood sugar, he started giving himself insulin injections at every meal. His doctor switched him to an external pump that delivers both a continuous (basal) dose and a bolus dose to cover mealtimes or other times to correct high blood sugar. Robert calls the pump "liberating" because he doesn't have to give himself injections with every meal, and his insulin dose is more precise. "The pump makes it easier for me to control my blood sugar. I love it," he says.

Implantable Insulin Pump. An implantable insulin pump is an insulin-delivery device surgically implanted under your skin. It delivers insulin in a way that mimics your body's own natural insulin production, even better than under-the-skin injections. The pump delivers a continuous basal dose of insulin through a catheter and into your abdominal cavity. You can self-administer a bolus dose with a remote-control device. These pumps are disk-shaped and weigh about 5 to 8 ounces.

Research into the effectiveness of implantable pumps shows that they may be associated with less variation in blood glucose levels and may result in fewer episodes of hypoglycemia than with multiple daily injections. In addition, patients using implantable pumps appear to be more satisfied with their treatment and did not gain weight as they had on an intensive self-injection regimen, according to one study. There can be complications, however, including blockage of the catheter and infection or other skin conditions at the implantation site. Despite the promise of these devices, these pumps are still used only experimentally in the United States and can be obtained only through participating in ongoing research studies.

Tools for the Visually Impaired

If you have vision problems, there are special devices designed to make injections easier for you. These include needle guides, which help you insert the needle into the correct insulin vial for drawing up an injection; syringe magnifiers that enlarge the measure marks on a syringe barrel; and nonvisual measurement tools that help you measure an accurate dose of insulin. There are countless other products available to make giving an injection seem effortless. The best source of information on insulin delivery is in the magazine *Diabetes Forecast*, which publishes a Resource Guide annually. You can also access the Resource Guide online at www.diabetes.org.

General Recommendations: Your Insulin Plan

Insulin plans generally employ one or two types of insulin and are designed to imitate the insulin secretion of a normal pancreas. Your doctor will give you instructions on how much you may need each day and will help you establish a personal insulin plan that suits your diet and lifestyle. Your insulin plan may include one dose as a basal insulin (generally given at night), two doses (generally given before breakfast and dinner), or multiple doses that involve premeal injections of a bolus insulin and an injection of long-acting insulin at night.

Ideally, you'll coordinate your insulin injections with your meals. Be sure to follow your doctor's guidelines explicitly on when to take your insulin. A rule of thumb is that you want insulin to begin working in your body at the same time your food is being absorbed. Referring to the "onset" column in the chart on page 219 can help you with the correct timing. Remember: "onset" tells you the approximate time when insulin starts to work in your body. Proper timing of insulin and meals will help avert low blood sugar levels.

There is an exception to these guidelines, however. Injections of long-acting insulins are not "timed" to meals because of their long duration of action. Also, you may need to take long-acting insulin with shorter-acting insulin products, depending on your individual situation, and you'll need to coordinate those insulins with your meals.

Monitoring Your Blood Sugar While on Insulin

With insulin, you'll need to check your blood sugar level regularly by using a blood glucose monitor (see Chapter 8). Your doctor or diabetes educator can teach you how to use the monitor. Write down each measurement, or retrieve the downloaded data from your meter, and show this record to your doctor, so he or she can tell you how much insulin to take and make adjustments if necessary.

The Future of Insulin Therapy

Several insulin products are in development, and there's no telling when they might become realities. You may have heard of inhaled insulin, marketed as Exubera. It was the first noninjectable insulin option introduced in the United States in more than eighty years. Exubera was an inhaled, rapid-acting, dry-powder form of insulin. It featured a portable inhaler for insulin, similar to the device used by people with asthma. With this system, insulin was provided as a dry powder, which was placed into an aerosol device for absorption by the lungs. You inhaled it through your mouth prior to each meal, thus absorbing the insulin in your lungs. The insulin that was absorbed through your lungs then went to work to help you metabolize glucose from your meals as would injected insulin. Unfortunately, Exubera was withdrawn from the market in 2007, not for reasons of safety or effectiveness, but because of a business decision made by the manufacturer. However, there are several other inhaled insulin formations under development, and the reports on these inhaled insulin products appear to be very favorable at this time. Thus, there is a good chance that an inhaled insulin may return to the market in the near future.

Scientists are also investigating "transdermal" insulin delivery systems—meaning "through the skin" in the form of skin patches. Patches have helped people quit smoking by delivering nicotine through the skin. Insulin, however, is a large molecule that is not readily absorbed through the skin, so there are challenges involved in the development of transdermal delivery of insulin. Nonetheless, scientists are working on patches using electrical currents, ultrasound waves, and chemicals to help transport insulin through the skin. These formulations are still considered many years away at this time.

Another line of investigation involves buccal (*BUCK-el*) insulin. It is similar to inhaled insulin in that it is taken through the mouth; however, it is sprayed into the mouth. Instead of going into the lungs, it is absorbed in the lining at the back of the mouth and throat. The drawback is that much of the insulin can be wasted and there are concerns with the variable absorption.

For decades, patients and doctors have hoped for insulin in pill form. But insulin taken as a pill is quickly broken down in the stomach, just like any food you'd eat. That makes it useless for restoring normal blood sugar levels. The research into this form of delivering insulin has focused on packaging the insulin using special coatings, or altering the insulin structure to get it through the stomach. Progress is being made, but it doesn't appear that we will have an oral insulin available any time soon.

Even so, there is much research energy being expended in prestigious laboratories all over the world in the development of new insulin technologies, and that alone should give you encouragement. But you should also remain encouraged that injected insulin (by syringe, pump, or pen) is truly an effective way to lower blood sugar levels. Even if one of the newer insulin delivery methods is not available for some time, rest assured that even today you can adequately control your diabetes with injections with minimal pain and inconvenience. No matter how you look at it, insulin is a powerfully effective drug that can allow you to control your blood sugar on a meal-to-meal and day-to-day basis to achieve a normal lifestyle and, most important, be put on a path to markedly reduce the chances of developing complications.

ASK DR. CEFALU: THERE ARE SO MANY DIABETES PRODUCTS ON THE MARKET. HOW DO I KNOW WHICH ONES ARE RIGHT FOR ME?

Many ads make a new diabetes product sound like it will work for everyone, but in fact it may only be useful for specific conditions. Your doctor, diabetes educator, and other members of your health-care team may have information on new products, and you should check with them when something new comes on the market. They will help you decide whether the new product is one you should try.

✳

ASK DR. CEFALU: ARE THERE FREE OR LOW-COST DIABETES COVERAGES AND SERVICES I CAN USE?

Yes. Here are some sources: the Bureau of Primary Health Care within the Health Resources and Services Administration (HRSA) has a nationwide network of community-based health-care centers that provides primary health-care services at little or no cost; access information at bphc.hrsa.gov. Hospitals and other health-care facilities participating in HRSA's Hill-Burton program provide free and low-cost services to eligible individuals. The Partnership for Prescription Assistance provides information about public and private patient assistance programs, which help low-income, uninsured patients get free or nearly free brand-name medicines; visit its Web site at www.pparx.org, or call 1-888-477-2669. You may also want to contact the American Diabetes Association for additional information.

✳

Appendix A

A1c. An important test that measures your average blood glucose level over the past two to three months. A1c is the technical name for a component (A1c) of hemoglobin in red blood cells. Blood sugar binds to hemoglobin and stays bound for the life of the cell, which is around three months. By measuring the amount of blood sugar bound to your hemoglobin, laboratory technicians can get a very good reading of your average blood sugar levels for the past three months.

Aerobic exercise. Continuous action exercise that requires the heart and lungs to work hard to meet the muscles' continuous demand for oxygen. Examples include walking, jogging, running, cycling, swimming, and cross-country skiing.

Albuminuria. A condition in which the urine contains more than normal amounts of a protein called albumin. Albuminuria suggests damage to the filtering system of the kidney and is an early sign of kidney disease.

Alpha cell. A type of cell in the pancreas that makes and releases a hormone called glucagon. Glucagon is a hormone that is secreted to help maintain glucose levels and is an important hormone needed by the body when blood glucose falls too low.

Alpha-glucosidase inhibitors. Oral diabetes agents that reduce blood glucose levels by blocking the enzymes that digest starch in the intestines. The net effect is a slower and lower rise in blood glucose throughout the day after meals.

Amino acids. Basic building blocks of protein necessary for growth and metabolism.

Amylin. A hormone made by beta cells in the pancreas that regulates glucose release into the bloodstream after eating and by slowing the emptying of the stomach.

Antioxidant. A special class of nutrients that fight free radicals, unstable molecules that damage otherwise healthy cells.

Atherosclerosis. The clogging, narrowing, and hardening of the body's large arteries and medium-size blood vessels. Atherosclerosis can lead to stroke, heart attack, and kidney disease.

Autonomic neuropathy. Diabetes-related nerve disease that can affect the lungs, heart, stomach, intestines, bladder, or genitals.

Beta cell. The insulin-producing cells of the pancreas. Beta cells are located in the islets of the pancreas.

Biguanide. A class of oral medicine used to treat type 2 diabetes, which lowers blood glucose by reducing the amount of glucose produced by the liver and by helping the body respond better to insulin.

Blood glucose. The main sugar found in the blood and the body's main source of energy. Also called blood sugar.

Blood glucose level. The amount of glucose in a given amount of blood. It is noted in milligrams per deciliter, or mg/dl.

Blood glucose meter. A small, portable machine used to check blood glucose levels. After pricking the skin with a lancet (small, thin needle), you place a droplet of blood on a test strip in the machine. The meter displays the blood glucose level as a number on the meter's digital readout.

Blood glucose monitoring. The process of checking your blood glucose level on a regular basis in order to manage diabetes.

Blood pressure. The force of blood exerted on the inside walls of blood vessels. Blood pressure is expressed as a ratio (example: 120/80, read as "120 over 80"). The first number is the systolic pressure, or the pressure when the heart pushes blood out into the arteries. The second number is the diastolic pressure, or the pressure when the heart rests.

Body mass index (BMI). A measurement used to evaluate body weight relative to your height. BMI is used to find out if you are underweight, normal weight, overweight, or obese.

Bolus. An extra amount of insulin taken to cover an expected rise in blood glucose, often related to a meal or snack.

Calories. Units that represent the amount of energy provided by food.

Carbohydrate. One of the three main nutrients in food. Carbohydrates are the body's main source of fuel. Foods that provide carbohydrate are starches, vegetables, fruits, dairy products, and sugars.

Carbohydrate counting. A method of meal planning for people with diabetes based on counting the number of grams of carbohydrate in food.

Cardiovascular disease. Disease of the heart and blood vessels, including conditions such as heart disease and stroke.

Cataract. An eye disease in which the lens of the eye becomes clouded.

Catheter. A thin, flexible tube that is inserted into a blood vessel or the body to provide a passageway, or to withdraw or inject fluids.

Certified diabetes educator (CDE). A health-care professional with expertise in diabetes. A CDE has met eligibility requirements and successfully completed a certification exam.

Cholesterol. A fatty substance found in some foods and manufactured by the body for many vital functions. Excess cholesterol and saturated fat can increase blood levels of cholesterol and can collect inside artery walls. This process contributes to heart disease.

Combination oral medicines. A pill that includes two or more different medicines.

Combination therapy. The use of different medicines together (oral diabetes agents or an oral diabetes agent and insulin) to manage the blood glucose levels of people with type 2 diabetes.

Complications. Serious effects of diabetes such as damage to the eyes, heart, blood vessels, nervous system, or kidneys.

Coronary heart disease. Heart disease caused by narrowing of the arteries that surround the heart, and supply blood to it. If the blood supply is cut off, the result is a heart attack.

Creatinine. A waste product from protein in the diet and from the muscles of the body. Creatinine is removed from the body by the kidneys; as kidney disease progresses, the level of creatinine in the blood increases.

Diabetes Control and Complications Trial (DCCT). A study by the National Institute of Diabetes and Digestive and Kidney Diseases conducted in people with type 1 diabetes. The study showed that intensive therapy compared to conventional therapy significantly helped prevent or delay diabetes complications. Intensive therapy included multiple daily insulin injections or the use of an insulin pump with multiple blood glucose readings each day.

Diabetes Prevention Program (DPP). A study by the National Institute of Diabetes and Digestive and Kidney Diseases conducted from 1998 to 2001 in people at high risk for type 2 diabetes. All study participants had prediabetes and were overweight. The study showed that people who lost 5 to 7 percent of their body weight through a low-fat, low-calorie diet and moderate exercise, e.g., usually walking for thirty minutes five days a week, reduced their risk of getting type 2 diabetes by 58 percent. Participants who received treatment with the oral diabetes drug metformin reduced their risk of getting type 2 diabetes by 31 percent.

Diabetic ketoacidosis (DKA). An emergency condition in which extremely high blood glucose levels, along with a severe lack of insulin, result in the breakdown of body fat for energy and an accumulation of ketones in the blood and urine. Signs of DKA are nausea and vomiting, stomach pain, fruity breath odor, and rapid breathing. Untreated, DKA can lead to coma and death.

Diabetic retinopathy. Diabetic eye disease in which there is damage to the small blood vessels in the retina. Loss of vision may result.

Dialysis. The process of cleaning wastes from the blood through artificial means. This job is normally done by the kidneys. If the kidneys fail, the blood must be cleaned artificially with special equipment.

Dietitian. A health-care professional who advises people about meal planning, weight control, and diabetes management. A registered dietitian (RD) has more training.

D-phenylalanine derivative. A new class of oral diabetes medications that releases insulin from your pancreas.

Endocrinologist. A physician who specializes in treating diseases of the glands and treats people with diabetes.

Fasting blood glucose test. A test of your blood glucose level after you have not eaten for eight to twelve hours (usually overnight). This test is used to diagnose prediabetes and diabetes. It is also used to monitor people with diabetes.

Fats. A food group that provides energy, but is the most concentrated source of calories in the diet. Examples of fats include margarine, butter, shortening, vegetable oils, salad dressings, and fish oils.

Fiber. The nondigestible portion of plants that may lower fat and glucose absorption and promote a healthy digestive system.

Gastroparesis. A form of neuropathy that affects the ability of the stomach to contract. Digestion of food may be incomplete or delayed, resulting in nausea, vomiting, or bloating, making blood glucose control difficult.

Gestational diabetes. A form of diabetes that develops during pregnancy and usually disappears upon delivery, but increases the risk that the mother will develop diabetes later.

Gingivitis. An inflammation of the gums characterized by redness and bleeding.

Glaucoma. An increase in fluid pressure inside the eye that may lead to loss of vision.

Glomerular filtration rate. A measure of the kidney's ability to filter and remove waste products from the body.

Glucagon. A hormone produced by the pancreas that raises blood glucose levels. An injectable form is available by prescription and used to treat a severe insulin reaction.

Glucose. Blood sugar. It acts as a fuel for the body.

Glucose tablets. Chewable tablets, available in pharmacies, made of pure glucose and used for treating hypoglycemia (low blood sugar).

Glucose tolerance. The ability to transport blood glucose into cells for use by the body.

Glycemic index of foods. A system of rating foods according to how fast they elevate blood glucose.

Glycogen. The form of carbohydrate found and stored in the liver and muscles.

Glycosuria. Glucose in the urine.

HDL (high-density lipoprotein). A type of cholesterol in the blood that has a protective effect against the buildup of plaque in the arteries.

Hemoglobin. The oxygen-carrying protein in red blood cells.

Hormone. A chemical produced in one part of the body and released into the blood to trigger or regulate particular functions of the body.

Hormone replacement therapy. The use of synthetic or natural hormones to treat a disease or a hormone deficiency. For example, the female hormones estrogen and progesterone are sometimes used to treat the symptoms of menopause.

Hyperglycemia. A condition in which blood glucose levels are too high.

Hypertension. High blood pressure. It occurs when blood flows through the blood vessels with a force greater than normal.

Hypoglycemia. A condition in which blood glucose levels drop too low, for example, in the range of 70 mg/dl or lower. Also called insulin reaction.

Immune system. A complex network of various types of cells and organs that work together to fight disease, from the common cold to cancers.

Impaired-fasting glucose (IFG). A condition in which a blood glucose test, taken after an eight- to twelve-hour fast, shows a level of glucose higher than normal but not high enough for a diagnosis of diabetes. IFG is a fasting glucose level of 100 mg/dl to 125 mg/dl.

Impaired glucose tolerance (IGT). The inability of the body to properly break down and use glucose. IGT often precedes type 2 diabetes and is a risk factor for the disease. A glucose tolerance test can detect IGT.

Implantable continuous glucose monitor. A system of glucose monitoring inserted under your skin to give you continuous measurements and readings of your glucose levels.

Implantable insulin pump. A small pump placed inside the body to deliver insulin in response to remote-control commands from the user.

Impotence. Inability to have or sustain an erection of the penis. Often a result of nerve (neuropathy) diabetes.

Inhaled insulin. A new treatment for taking insulin using a portable device that allows you to breathe in insulin. The insulin is absorbed through the lungs.

Injection sites. Places on the body where insulin is usually injected.

Insulin. A hormone that decreases blood glucose levels by moving glucose into cells to be used for fuel.

Insulin adjustment. A change in the amount of insulin a person with diabetes takes based on factors such as meal planning, activity, and blood glucose levels.

Insulin pen. A device for injecting insulin that resembles a fountain pen and holds replaceable cartridges of insulin.

Insulin pump. A device that delivers a steady release of insulin (basal dose) but can also deliver a large dose prior to meals (bolus dose).

Insulin reaction. Low blood sugar as a result of too much insulin, either injected or from your own body, for the amount of food or exercise.

Insulin receptors. Areas on the outer part of a cell that allow the cell to attach to insulin in the blood. When the cell and insulin bind, the cell can take in glucose from the blood and use it for energy.

Insulin resistance. A condition in which the body does not respond to glucose properly and is associated with obesity and type 2 diabetes.

Intensive therapy. A treatment for diabetes in which blood glucose is kept as close to normal as possible through frequent injections (premeal fast-acting and basal coverage with long-acting insulin at night) or use of an insulin pump. Doses used in intensive insulin therapy may be adjusted based on carbohydrates consumed at each meal, exercise, and on blood glucose test results.

Intermediate-acting insulin. Insulin that reaches the bloodstream about two to four hours after it is injected, peaks four to twelve hours later, and may work up to eighteen hours.

Islet cells. Specialized cells in the pancreas that are arranged in clusters, or islets. Insulin is released from beta cells in the islets.

Jet injector. A device that uses high pressure instead of a needle to propel insulin through the skin and into the body.

Ketones. By-products of the breakdown of fat for fuel.

Ketonuria. A condition occurring when ketones are present in the urine, a warning sign of diabetic ketoacidosis.

Ketosis. A buildup of ketones in the body that may lead to diabetic ketoacidosis. Signs of ketosis are nausea, vomiting, and stomach pain.

Kidney failure. A chronic condition in which the body retains fluid, and harmful wastes build up, because the kidneys no longer work properly. A person with kidney failure needs dialysis or a kidney transplant. Also called end-stage renal disease, or ESRD.

Lactic acidosis. A rare but serious condition brought on by the buildup of lactic acid in the blood. Lactic acid is a waste product of glucose metabolism. Lactic acidosis can be fatal in many cases.

Lancet. The fine needle used to prick skin for a blood glucose test.

LDL cholesterol (low-density cholesterol). A type of cholesterol in the blood, known as the "bad" kind because it increases the risk of heart disease.

Lente insulin. An intermediate-acting insulin. On average, lente insulin starts to lower blood glucose levels within two to four hours after injection but keeps working for eighteen hours after injection.

Lipid. A term for fat in the body.

Lipid profile. A blood test that measures total cholesterol, triglycerides, LDL ("bad" cholesterol), and HDL ("good" cholesterol). This test is used as one measure of your cardiovascular risk.

Lispro insulin. A rapid-acting insulin. On average, lispro insulin starts to lower blood glucose within fifteen minutes after injection. It has its strongest effect sixty minutes after injection but keeps working for four to five hours after injection.

Macrovascular disease. Disease of the large blood vessels, such as those found in the heart.

Macula. The part of the retina in the eye used for reading and seeing fine detail.

Macular edema. A swelling of the macula, an area near the center of the retina that is responsible for fine or reading vision. Macular edema is a complication that may be associated with diabetic retinopathy.

Meglitinides. A class of oral medicine for type 2 diabetes, which lowers blood glucose by helping the pancreas release more insulin right after meals.

Metabolic rate. The rate at which the body burns calories.

Metabolic syndrome. A cluster of several conditions, including obesity, insulin resistance, diabetes or prediabetes, hypertension, and high lipids.

Metabolism. The physiological process that converts food to energy so that the body can function.

mg/dl. Stands for milligrams per deciliter and is a unit of measure that shows the concentration of a substance in a specific amount of fluid. In the United States, blood glucose test results are reported as mg/dl.

Microalbuminuria. The presence of small amounts of albumin, a protein, in the urine. Microalbuminuria is an early sign of kidney damage, or nephropathy, which is a common and serious complication of diabetes.

Microvascular disease. Disease of the smallest blood vessels, such as those found in the eyes, nerves, and kidneys.

Mineral. A class of nutrients found in foods and needed by the body for a wide range of enzymatic and metabolic functions. Examples include calcium, magnesium, and potassium.

Mixed dose. A combination of two types of insulin in one injection. Usually a rapid- or short-acting insulin is combined with a longer-acting insulin (such as NPH insulin) to provide both short-term and long-term control of blood glucose levels.

Monounsaturated fat. Fatty acids that lack two hydrogen atoms. Found in such foods as olive oil, olives, avocados, cashew nuts, and cold-water fish such as salmon, mackerel, halibut, and swordfish.

Nephrologist. A physician who specializes in treating people with kidney problems.

Nephropathy. A disease of the kidneys that can be caused by high blood glucose and high blood pressure.

Neurologist. A physician who specializes in treating problems of the nervous system.

Neuropathy. Nerve disease.

Noninvasive blood glucose monitoring. A way to measure your blood glucose without pricking your finger to obtain a blood sample.

NPH insulin. An intermediate-acting insulin; NPH stands for neutral protamine Hagedorn. On average, NPH insulin starts to lower blood glucose within two to four hours after injection. It has its strongest effect four to six hours after injection but keeps working about twelve to sixteen hours after injection.

Obesity. A condition in which a greater than normal amount of fat is in the body; more severe than overweight; having a body mass index (BMI) of 30 or more.

Ophthalmologist. A medical doctor who diagnoses and treats eye diseases and eye disorders. Opthalmologists can also prescribe glasses and contact lenses.

Oral diabetes agents. Medications taken by mouth that are designed to lower blood sugar. They are usually prescribed to people with type 2 diabetes and are not to be confused with insulin.

Oral glucose tolerance test (OGTT). A test to diagnose prediabetes and diabetes. After an overnight fast, a blood sample is taken, then you drink a high-glucose beverage. Blood samples are taken at intervals for two to three hours. Test results are compared with a standard and show how the body uses glucose over time.

Overweight. An above-normal body weight; usually having a body mass index (BMI) of 25 to 29.9.

Pancreas. A flask-shaped organ situated behind and just below the stomach. Its job is to secrete powerful digestive enzymes for the breakdown of food and to promote the production of insulin from beta cells in the pancreas.

Periodontal disease. Infection and damage to the gums. May be a complication of diabetes.

Peripheral neuropathy. Nerve damage that affects the feet, legs, or hands.

Pharmacist. A health-care professional who prepares and dispenses prescription medicine to people. Pharmacists can also provide information on medicines and how they interact with each other.

Photocoagulation. A treatment for diabetic retinopathy in which a laser seals off bleeding blood vessels in the eye.

Podiatrist. A doctor who treats foot problems and helps people keep their feet healthy by providing regular foot examinations and treatment.

Prediabetes. A condition in which blood glucose levels are higher than normal but are not high enough for a diagnosis of diabetes. People with prediabetes are at increased risk for developing type 2 diabetes and for heart disease and stroke.

Premixed insulin. A commercially produced combination of two different types of insulin.

Proliferative retinopathy. A condition in which new blood vessels grow along the retina and in the vitreous humor of the eye.

Protein. One of the three main nutrients in food. Food group necessary for growth and repair of body tissues. Examples include meat, poultry, fish, eggs, dairy products, legumes, nuts, and seeds.

Proteinuria. The presence of protein in the urine, indicating that the kidneys are not working properly.

Rapid-acting insulin. A type of insulin that starts to lower blood glucose within ten to fifteen minutes after injection and has its strongest effect approximately sixty minutes after injection.

Receptor. A physiological signal device located on the membrane of a cell. Receptors recognize substances such as hormones, nutrients, or drugs and allow access to the cell.

Regular insulin. A type of short-acting insulin. On average, regular insulin starts to lower blood glucose within thirty minutes after injection. It has its strongest effect two to four hours after injection but keeps working six to eight hours after injection.

Retina. The light-sensing part of the eye.

Retinopathy. Damage to tiny blood vessels in the eye that can lead to vision problems. Retinopathy is a severe complication of diabetes.

Saturated fat. A fatty acid that is solid at room temperature. Butter and other forms of animal fat are examples of saturated fat. An excess of saturated fat in the diet can raise the risk of heart disease.

Short-acting insulin. See regular insulin.

Side effect. The unintended action(s) of a drug.

Starch. A type of carbohydrate, one of the three main nutrients in food.

Strength training. Any kind of weight-bearing activity in which your muscles are challenged to work harder each time they're exercised.

Stress hormones. Hormones released when the body is under stress. Stress hormones include cortisol, adrenaline, and nonepinephrine.

Stroke. Condition caused by damage to blood vessels in the brain; may cause loss of ability to speak or to move parts of the body.

Subcutaneous injection. Injecting a fluid into the tissue under the skin with a needle and syringe.

Sugar. A form of carbohydrate that supplies calories and can elevate blood glucose levels.

Sugar substitutes. Sweeteners that can be used in place of sugar to reduce calories. Substitutes include saccharin, aspartame, acesulfame-K, and sugar alcohols.

Sulfonylureas. Oral diabetes medications that reduce blood glucose by stimulating the pancreas to produce more insulin.

Thiazolidinediones. A class of oral diabetes medications that reduce insulin resistance by making cells more sensitive to the body's own insulin.

Triglycerides. Fats that circulate in the blood until they are deposited in fat cells.

Type 1 diabetes. A form of diabetes that generally develops prior to age thirty but may occur at any age. It is caused by an immune system attack on the body's own beta cells. When these cells are destroyed, insulin can no longer be produced.

Type 2 diabetes. A form of diabetes that occurs generally in people over age forty but can develop at any age. Associated with obesity in the majority of cases. With type 2 diabetes, the body does not use insulin properly.

Unit of insulin. The basic measure of insulin. U-100 insulin means 100 units of insulin per milliliter (ml) or cubic centimeter (cc) of solution. Most insulin made today in the United States is U-100.

United Kingdom Prospective Diabetes Study (UKPDS). A large study in England conducted in people with type 2 diabetes. The study showed that if people lowered their blood sugar, they lowered their risk of eye disease and kidney damage. In addition, those with type 2 diabetes and hypertension who lowered their blood pressure also reduced their risk of stroke, eye damage, and death from long-term complications.

Urine tests. Tests that measure substances in the urine, including ketones.

Vitamins. Organic substances found in food that perform many vital functions in the body.

Vitrectomy. Surgery that improves sight by removing the cloudy vitreous humor in the eye and replaces it with a salt solution.

Vitreous humor. The clear gel that lies behind the eye's lens and in front of the retina.

Appendix B

Stretching Exercises and Guidelines

How to Stretch

- Do a short warm-up such as walking or marching in place *before* stretching.
- Move slowly until you feel the muscle stretch. A safe stretch is gentle and relaxing.
- Hold the stretch steady for fifteen to thirty seconds. Do NOT bounce.
- Relax. Then repeat three to five times.
- Stretch within your own limits. Don't compete.
- Breathe slowly and naturally. Do NOT hold your breath.
- Relax, enjoy, and feel good about yourself.

Important: Never stretch if you have pain before you begin. If a particular stretch causes pain, stop doing it. *Listen to your body!*

Here are some safe and easy stretches:

1. Arm Reaches

- Stand up straight with your feet shoulder-width apart.
- Counting to five, stretch your right arm to the ceiling while keeping your feet flat on the floor. Repeat with your left arm.
- Do this ten times. When finished, shake out your arms.

2. Arm Circles

- Stand with feet shoulder-width apart, knees slightly bent.
- Extend your arms straight out from the shoulders with your fingers spread and palms down. Keep your buttocks and stomach tight.
- Rotate your arms in circles ten times forward and then ten times backward. When finished, shake out your arms.
- Over time work up to twenty circles in each direction.

3. Waist Bends

- Stand up tall with your feet shoulder-width apart.
- Bend to the right, bringing your right arm down the side of your body and left arm over your head. Look straight ahead and count to ten. Slowly return to the straight-up position.
- Repeat the exercise, bending to the left side.
- Over time work up to five of these.

4. Sitting Toe Touch

- Sit on the floor with your feet placed flat against a wall, knees slightly bent. Reach out your hands and slowly stretch them toward your toes. Keep breathing.
- Repeat two or three times to start.
- Over time work your way up to ten of these.

5. Back Press

- Lie on your back with your knees bent and your hands clasped behind your neck. Keep your feet flat on the floor. Take a deep breath and relax.
- Press the small of your back against the floor and tighten your stomach and buttock muscles. This should cause the lower end of the pelvis to rotate forward and flatten your back against the floor.
- Hold for five seconds. Relax.

6. Back Stretch

- Lie on your back with your knees bent and your arms flat on the floor at your sides. Keep your feet flat on the floor. Take a deep breath and relax.
- Grasp the back of one knee (*not* the top of the knee) with both hands and pull as close to your chest as possible. Return to the starting position.
- Repeat with the other leg.

7. Heel Cord (Achilles) Stretch

- Stand facing a wall an arm's distance away, with your knees straight and your heels flat on the floor.
- With your hands resting on the wall, allow your body to lean forward by bending your elbows slowly. Keep your legs and body straight and your heels on the floor.

8. Calf Stretch

- Stand straight with feet shoulder-width apart.
- Step forward with your right foot, slightly bending your right knee. The front of your knee should be lined up with the front of your toes. Your left leg should stay relatively straight and your left heel should remain on the floor. Hold for ten to twenty seconds.
- Slightly bend your left knee. Hold for ten to twenty seconds.
- Repeat for the opposite side.

If you do get a sprain, strain, "pull," or bruise, apply the R.I.C.E. technique:

Rest (restrict movement)

- Stop doing the activity.
- Rest for a few days. This will promote healing.
- Sometimes splints, tapes, or bandages are necessary.

Ice

- Apply ice or cold compresses for the first twenty-four to thirty-six hours after the injury. This reduces pain, bleeding, and swelling. Have your doctor evaluate the condition.
- Schedule: ten minutes on, ten minutes off.

- *Always* wrap ice or compresses in an absorbent towel or cloth. Don't apply directly or wrapped in plastic—that can cause frostbite and more injury.

Compression (pressure)

- Apply pressure by wrapping the injury with an elastic bandage. This helps to reduce swelling and blood flow to the area.
- The bandage should be tight enough to reduce blood flow but not cut it off completely. Loosen the bandage if your toes or fingers begin to feel numb or lose their color.

Elevation

- Lift the injured area above heart level. Keep it elevated whenever possible, not just during icing.
- This helps reduce internal bleeding and pooling of blood in the area that can cause pain and throbbing.

Appendix C

[## Resources]

For additional information, here are key organizations that can provide you with additional information and support on diabetes.

American Association of Diabetes Educators (AADE)
100 West Monroe Street
Suite 400
Chicago, IL 60603
800-338-3633
www.aadenet.org
   A professional organization that helps you locate a diabetes educator in your community.

American Diabetes Association (ADA)
Attn: National Call Center
1701 North Beauregard Street
Alexandria, VA 22311
800-DIABETES (800-342-2383)
www.diabetes.org

The American Diabetes Association is considered the leading authority for information on diabetes education and treatment. The ADA publishes books and resources for providers and people with diabetes, including *Diabetes Forecast,* a monthly magazine for patients, and the journals *Diabetes* and *Diabetes Care* for the health professional.

American Dietetic Association
120 South Riverside Plaza
Suite 2000
Chicago, IL 60606-6995
800-877-1600
www.eatright.org

A professional organization that can help you locate a registered dietitian in your community.

American Heart Association
7272 Greenville Avenue
Dallas, TX 75231
800-AHA-USA-1 (800-242-8721)
www.americanheart.org

A private, voluntary organization that distributes literature on heart disease and its prevention. Local affiliates can be found in the telephone directory.

American Optometric Association
1505 Prince Street
Suite 300
Alexandria, VA 22314
800-365-2219
www.aoanet.org

A federation of state, student, and armed forces optometric associations that can help you find an optometrist in your area.

American Podiatric Medical Association
9312 Old Georgetown Road
Bethesda, MD 20814
301-571-9200 or 800-ASK-APMA
www.apma.org

APMA publishes materials for professionals and the public, and can help you locate a podiatrist in your area.

Amputee Resource Foundation of America, Inc.
2324 Wildwood Trail
Minnetonka, MN 55305
e-mail: info@amputeeresource.org
www.amputeeresource.org
    Disseminates useful information, performs charitable services, and conducts research to enhance productivity and quality of life for amputees in America.

Department of Veterans Affairs
www.va.gov/diabetes
    Information for providers and veterans on diabetes care.

Diabetes Exercise & Sports Association (DESA)
8001 Montcastle Drive
Nashville, TN 37221
800-898-4322
www.diabetes-exercise.org
    Provides pamphlets on diabetes and exercise.

Health Resources and Services Administration
www.hrsa.gov
    The primary federal agency for improving access to health-care services for people who are uninsured, isolated, or medically vulnerable.

Indian Health Service (IHS)
The Reyes Building
801 Thompson Avenue
Suite 400
Rockville, MD 20852-1627
301-443-1083
www.ihs.gov
    Provides information tailored to Native American and Alaska Native communities, general diabetes information, nutrition, educational materials, and professional resources.

International Association for Medical Assistance to Travelers (IAMAT)
1623 Military Road #279
Niagara Falls, NY 14304-1745
716-754-4883
www.iamat.org
Can provide a list of doctors in foreign countries who can speak English and were trained either in North America or Great Britain.

International Diabetes Federation (IDF)
Avenue Emile De Mot 19
B-1000 Brussels, Belgium
011+32-2-53855111
www.idf.org
The International Diabetes Federation (IDF) is a worldwide alliance of over 200 diabetes associations in more than 160 countries, who have come together to enhance the lives of people with diabetes everywhere. For over 50 years, IDF has been at the vanguard of global diabetes advocacy.

Joslin Diabetes Center
One Joslin Place
Boston, MA 02215
617-732-2400
www.joslin.org
The Joslin Diabetes Center is an international leader in diabetes research, treatment, and patient and professional education. It is affiliated with Harvard Medical School.

Juvenile Diabetes Foundation (JDF) International
120 Wall Street
New York, NY 10005-4001
800-533-CURE (800-533-2873)
www.jdrf.org
A private, voluntary organization that funds research on diabetes and promotes public awareness. Local chapters located across the country sponsor program and fund-raising activities. Information about local groups is available in telephone directories or from the national office.

Medic Alert Foundation
2323 Colorado Avenue
Turlock, CA 95382
888-633-4298; 209-668-3333 from outside the U.S.
www.medicalert.org

Supplies medical ID bracelets and maintains a twenty-four-hour emergency response center to respond to calls regarding members.

National Diabetes Education Program (NDEP)
800-CDC-INFO (800-232-4636); 888-232-6348 TTY
e-mail: cdcinfo@cdc.gov
www.cdc.gov/diabetes/ndep/index.htm

Joint program of CDC, the National Institutes of Health, and two hundred–plus partners; partners work together to improve the treatment and outcome of diabetes in individuals, families, communities, and health-care systems.

National Eye Institute (NEI)
National Eye Health Education Program
2020 Vision Place
Bethesda, MD 20892
301-496-5248
www.nei.nih.gov

Provides materials related to diabetic eye disease and its treatment, including literature for patients, guides for health-care professionals, and education kits for health-care workers and pharmacists.

National Institute of Diabetes and Digestive and Kidney Diseases (NIDDK)
Office of Communications & Public Liaison
Building 31, Room 9A06
31 Center Drive, MSC 2560
Bethesda, MD 20892-2560
301-496-3583
www.niddk.nih.gov

Conducts and supports research on many of the most serious diseases affecting public health, such as diabetes, endocrine disorders, digestive diseases, nutrition, urology, and renal disease.

National Kidney Foundation
30 East 33rd Street
New York, NY 10016
800-622-9010
www.kidney.org

A voluntary health organization that seeks to prevent kidney and urinary tract diseases, improve the health and well-being of individuals and families affected by these diseases, and increase the availability of all organs for transplantation.

Office of Minority Health Resource Center
Office of the Director
The Tower Building
1101 Wootton Parkway
Suite 600
Rockville, MD 20852
800-444-6472; 240-453-2882
www.omhrc.gov

Offers information, publications, and referrals to African-American, Asian, Hispanic/Latino, Native American/Alaska Native, and Pacific Islander populations.

Pedorthic Footwear Association
2025 M Street, NW
Suite 800
Washington, DC 20036
202-367-1145; 800-673-8447
www.pedorthics.org

Provides information on Medicare coverage of therapeutic shoes for people with diabetes.

Weight Control Information Network (WIN)
1 WIN Way
Bethesda, MD 20892-3665
877-946-4627
win.niddk.nih.gov/index.htm

A service of NIDDK. Provides fact sheets, pamphlets, reprints, consensus statements, reports, and literature searches on weight control, obesity, and weight-related nutritional disorders.

Appendix D

[**References**]

CHAPTER 1: UNDERSTANDING DIABETES AND HOW WE CAN STOP IT

The Diabetes Control and Complications Trial Research Group. 1993. The effect of intensive treatment of diabetes on the development and progression of long-term complications in insulin-dependent diabetes mellitus. *The New England Journal of Medicine* 329:977–986.

The Diabetes Control and Complications Trial Research Group. 2005. The diabetes control and complications trial/epidemiology of diabetes interventions and complications (EDIC) research group. Intensive diabetes treatment and cardiovascular disease in patients with type 1 diabetes. *The New England Journal of Medicine* 353:2643–2653.

Diabetes Prevention Program Research Group. 2002. Reduction in the incidence of type 2 diabetes with lifestyle intervention or metformin. *The New England Journal of Medicine* 346:393–403.

United Kingdom Prospective Diabetes Study (UKPDS) Group. 1998. Intensive blood-glucose control with sulphonylureas or insulin compared with conventional treatment and risk of complications in patients with type 2 diabetes. *The Lancet* 352:837–853.

CHAPTER 2: BEWARE OF METABOLIC SYNDROME AND PREDIABETES

American Diabetes Association. 2007. Standards of Medical Care in Diabetes— 2007. *Diabetes Care* 30:S3.

Buchanan, T. A., Xiang, A. H., Peters, R. K., et al. 2002. Preservation of pancreatic B-cell function and prevention of type 2 diabetes by pharmacological treatment of insulin resistance in high-risk Hispanic women. *Diabetes* 51:2769–2803.

Diabetes Prevention Program Research Group. 2002. Reduction in the incidence of type 2 diabetes with lifestyle intervention or metformin. *The New England Journal of Medicine* 346:393–403.

The DREAM Trial Investigators. 2006. Effect of rosiglitazone on the frequency of diabetes in patients with impaired glucose tolerance or impaired-fasting glucose: a randomized controlled trial. *The Lancet* 368:1096–1105.

Lakka, H. M., Laaksonen, D. E., Lakka, T. A., et al. 2002. The metabolic syndrome and total and cardiovascular disease mortality in middle-aged men. *The Journal of the American Medical Association* 288:2709–2716.

Lakka, H. M., Lakka, T. A., et al. 2002. Abdominal obesity is associated with increased risk of acute coronary events in men. *European Heart Journal* 23:706–713.

Tuomilehto, J., Lindstrom, J., Eriksson, J. G., et al. 2001. Prevention of type 2 diabetes mellitus by changes in lifestyle among subjects with impaired glucose tolerance. *The New England Journal of Medicine* 344:1343–1350.

CHAPTER 3: THE GOOD AND BAD NEWS ABOUT COMPLICATIONS

American Diabetes Association. 2007. Standards of Medical Care in Diabetes—2007. *Diabetes Care* 30:S3.

The Diabetes Control and Complications Trial Research Group. 2005. The diabetes control and complications trial/epidemiology of diabetes interventions and complications (EDIC) research group. Intensive diabetes treatment and cardiovascular disease in patients with type 1 diabetes. *The New England Journal of Medicine* 353: 2643–2653.

Perkins, B. A., Ficociello, L. H., Silva, K. H., et al. 2003. Regression of microalbuminuria in type 1 diabetes. *The New England Journal of Medicine* 348:2285–2293.

United Kingdom Prospective Diabetes Study (UKPDS) Group. 1998. Intensive blood-glucose control with sulphonylureas or insulin compared with conventional treatment and risk of complications in patients with type 2 diabetes. *The Lancet* 352:837–853.

CHAPTER 4: MAKING THE MOST OF YOUR FOOD

American Diabetes Association. 2007. Standards of Medical Care in Diabetes—2007. *Diabetes Care* 30:S3.

Browning, L. M., and Jebb, S. A. 2006. Nutritional influences on inflammation and type 2 diabetes risk. *Diabetes Technology and Therapeutics* 8:45–54.

Burani, J., and Longo, P. J. 2006. Low-glycemic index carbohydrates: an effective behavioral change for glycemic control and weight management in patients with type 1 and type 2 diabetes. *The Diabetes Educator* 32:78–88.

Ditschuneit, H. H. 2006. Do meal replacement drinks have a role in diabetes management? *Nestle Nutritional Workshop* 11:171–179.

CHAPTER 6: THE PROMISE OF COMPLEMENTARY THERAPY

Barringer, T. A., Kirk, J. K., Santaniello, A. C., et al. 2003. Effect of a multivitamin and mineral supplement on infection and quality of life. A randomized, double-blind, placebo-controlled trial. *Annals of Internal Medicine* 138:365–371.

Cefalu, W. T., and Hu, F. B. 2004. Chromium in human health. *Diabetes Care* 27:2741–2751.

Dham, S., et al. 2006. The role of complementary and alternative medicine in diabetes. *Current Diabetes Reports* 6:251–258.

Evans, J. L. 2003. Diet, botanical, and nutritional treatments for type 2 diabetes. Endotext.com

Foster, T. S. 2007. Efficacy and safety of alpha-lipoic acid supplementation in the treatment of symptomatic diabetic neuropathy. *Diabetes Educator* 33:111–117.

Hooper, P. L. 1999. Hot-tub therapy for type 2 diabetes mellitus. *The New England Journal of Medicine* 341:924–925.

Kleefstra, N., et al. 2006. Chromium treatment has no effect in patients with poorly controlled, insulin-treated type 2 diabetes in an obese Western population: a randomized, double-blind, placebo-controlled trial. *Diabetes Care* 29:521–525.

Lonn, E., Bosch, J., Yusuf, S., et al. 2005. Effects of long-term vitamin E supplementation on cardiovascular events and cancer: a randomized controlled trial. *The Journal of the American Medical Association* 293(11):1338–1347.

McGinnis, R. A., McGrady, A., Cox, S. A., et al. 2005. Biofeedback-assisted relaxation in type 2 diabetes. *Diabetes Care* 28:2145–2149.

Mossman, J. 2005. Dietary Supplements for Diabetes. *U.S. Pharmacist* 11:86–91.

Ribnicky, D. M., Poulev, A., Watford, M., Cefalu, W. T., et al. 2006. Antihyperglycemic activity of Tarralin, an ethanolic extract of Artemisia dracunculus L. *Phytomedicine* 13:550–557.

Ribnicky, D. M., Poulev, A., O'Neal, J., et al. 2004. Toxicological evaluation of the ethanolic extract of Artemisia dracunculus L. for use as a dietary supplement and in functional foods. *Food and Chemical Toxicology* 42:585–598.

Yeh, G. Y., et al. 2003. Systematic review of herbs and dietary supplements for glycemic control in diabetes. *Diabetes Care* 26:1277–1294.

CHAPTER 7: EXERCISING YOUR OPTIONS

American Diabetes Association. 2007. Standards of Medical Care in Diabetes—2007. *Diabetes Care* 30:S3.

Diabetes Prevention Program Research Group. 2002. Reduction in the incidence of type 2 diabetes with lifestyle intervention or metformin. *The New England Journal of Medicine* 346:393–403.

Rooney, B., et al. Is knowing enough? Increasing physical activity by wearing a pedometer. *Wisconsin Medical Journal* 102:31–36.

Warburton, D. E. R., et al. 2006. Prescribing exercise as preventive therapy. *Canadian Medical Association Journal* 174:961–974.

CHAPTER 8: GLUCOSE TESTING MADE PAIN-FREE AND EASY

American Diabetes Association. 2007. Standards of Medical Care in Diabetes–2007. *Diabetes Care* 30:S3.

The Diabetes Control and Complications Trial Research Group. 2005. The diabetes control and complications trial/epidemiology of diabetes interventions and complications (EDIC) research group. Intensive diabetes treatment and cardiovascular disease in patients with type 1 diabetes. *The New England Journal of Medicine* 353:2643–2653.

United Kingdom Prospective Diabetes Study (UKPDS) Group. 1998. Intensive blood-glucose control with sulphonylureas or insulin compared with conventional treatment and risk of complications in patients with type 2 diabetes. *The Lancet* 352:837–853.

CHAPTER 9: KEEPING THE MOMENTUM: REAP THE BENEFITS OF OUTSIDE SUPPORT

Diabetes Prevention Program Research Group. 2002. Reduction in the incidence of type 2 diabetes with lifestyle intervention or metformin. *The New England Journal of Medicine* 346:393–403.

McMahon, G. T., Gomes, H. E., et al. 2005. Web-based care management in patients with poorly controlled diabetes. *Diabetes Care* 28:1624–1629.

CHAPTER 10: OPTIMIZING YOUR ANTIDIABETES MEDICATIONS

American Diabetes Association. 2007. Standards of Medical Care in Diabetes— 2007. *Diabetes Care* 30:S3.

Cefalu, W. T. 2001. The use of hormone replacement therapy in postmenopausal women with type 2 diabetes. *Journal of Women's Health and Gender-Based Medicine* 10(3):241–255.

Green, B. D., Flatt, P. R., and Bailey, C. J. 2006. Dipeptidyl peptidase IV (DPP-IV) inhibitors: a newly emerging drug class for the treatment of type 2 diabetes. *Diabetes & Vascular Disease Research* 3:159–165.

CHAPTER 11: USING INSULIN: NOT THE PAIN IT USED TO BE

Cappelleri, J. C., Cefalu, W. T., Rosenstock, J., et al. 2002. Treatment satisfaction in type 2 diabetes: a comparison between an inhaled insulin regimen and a subcutaneous insulin regimen. *Clinical Therapeutics* 24:552–564.

DeFronzo, R. A., Bergenstal, R. M., Cefalu, W. T., et al. 2005. Efficacy of inhaled insulin in patients with type 2 diabetes not controlled with diet and exercise. *Diabetes Care* 28:1922–1928.

Rosenstock, J., Zinman, B., Cefalu, W. T., et al. 2005. Inhaled insulin improves glycemic control when substituted for or added to oral combination therapy in type 2 diabetes: a randomized, controlled trial. *Annals of Internal Medicine* 143: 549–558.

Skyler, J. S., Cefalu, W. T., Kourides, I. A., et al. 2001. Efficacy of inhaled human insulin in type 1 diabetes mellitus: a randomized proof-of-concept study. *The Lancet* 357:331–335.

Index

A1c (glycated hemoglobin test), 3, 37, 184–85, 214
abdominal fat, 22–23, 165
acarbose (Precose), 208
ACCORD (Action to Control Cardiovascular Risk in Diabetes), 3, 182
ACE (angiotensin converting enzymes) inhibitors, 45, 53
Actoplus Met (pioglitazone + metformin), 208
Actos (pioglitazone), 208–9
acupuncture, 153
adjunctive therapies. See complementary and alternative medicine (CAM)
adult onset diabetes (type 2), 11–13, 14–15, 16–18
aerobic exercise, 161–63
alcohol consumption, 84
aloe vera supplements, 150–51
alpha-blockers, 54
alpha lipoic acid supplements, 144
alpha-glucosidase inhibitors, 207–8

alternative medicine. See complementary and alternative medicine (CAM)
Amaryl (glimepiride), 205
American Association of Diabetes Educators, Web address, 190
American Diabetes Association, contact information, 189
American Dietetic Association, Web address, 191
Anderson, Richard, 138
anticonvulsants, 47
ARBs (angiotensin receptor blockers), 45, 53
artificial sweeteners, 85
aspirin, 51, 144
Avandamet (rosiglitazone + metformin), 208–9
Avandaryl (rosiglitazone + glimepiride), 208
Avandia (rosiglitazone), 32, 208–9

beta-blockers, 53–54
biguanides, 207

bile acid resins, 50
biofeedback, 153–54
bitter melon supplements, 146
blindness due to retinopathy, 40–44
blood glucose. *See* blood sugar; blood sugar
   testing
blood lipids. *See* cholesterol levels
blood pressure, high. *See* hypertension
blood sugar
   carbohydrate counting, 82–83
   chromium supplements and, 138
   control of, for management of complica-
      tions, 10–11, 33, 36
   in diagnosis of metabolic syndrome, 23
   diet and, 61–62
   exercise and, 157–58
   insulin and, 12
   integrated approach to control of, 11–12,
      15
   target range, 3, 182
blood sugar testing
   A1c (glycated hemoglobin test), 3, 37,
      184–85, 214
   equipment maintenance, 182–83
   fasting blood glucose test, 24, 29–30, 37,
      182
   during illness, 184, 186
   implantable continuous glucose moni-
      tors, 179–81
   during insulin therapy, 223
   laser tool for, 181–82
   new systems, 179–82
   oral glucose tolerance test (OGTT),
      24–25
   record keeping, 223
   self-monitoring (SMBG), 177–78
   target range, 182
   traditional systems, 178–79
   urine testing, 183–84
   value of, 175–78
blood thinners, drug interactions with, 153
blood vessel diseases. *See* vascular diseases
botanical extract supplements
   aloe vera, 150–51
   bitter melon, 146
   efficacy of, 145–46
   fenugreek, 147
   garlic, 152–53
   ginseng, 150
   gymnema sylvestre, 147–48
   ivy gourd, 148–49
   nopal (prickly pear cactus), 149
   Russian tarragon (Tarralin), 151–52
Byetta (exenatide), 210–11

calcium channel blockers, 54
calories
   diet foods, 86
   meal replacements, 87–89
   weight loss and, 73–74
CAM. *See* complementary and alternative
   medicine (CAM)
carbohydrates
   carbohydrate counting, 82–83
   fiber-rich, 64–66
   glycemic index, 86–87
cardiometabolic risk, 22
cardiovascular disease. *See* heart disease;
   vascular diseases
chlorpropamide (Diabinese), 205
cholesterol levels
   cardiovascular disease risk, 48–49, 57
   cholesterol-lowering drugs, 50, 135
   dietary cholesterol intake and, 68
   dietary fats and, 67–68
   exercise and, 159
   fasting lipid profile, 38, 39
   in metabolic syndrome, 22–23
   niacin supplements and, 135
   target levels, 38, 39, 47, 48–49
chromium supplements, 136–39
coenzyme Q_{10} supplements, 145
combination drug therapy, 212–13
complementary and alternative medicine
   (CAM)
   acupuncture, 153
   adjunctive therapies, definition of,
      132–33
   aloe vera, 150–51
   alpha lipoic acid, 144
   biofeedback, 153–54
   bitter melon, 146
   botanical extracts, 145–53
   chromium, 136–39
   coenzyme Q_{10}, 145
   definition of, 133
   Dietary Reference Intakes (DRIs),
      131–32
   drug interactions, 135, 141, 144, 153, 216
   fenugreek, 147
   garlic, 152–53
   ginseng, 150
   gymnema sylvestre, 147–48
   ivy gourd, 148–49
   magnesium, 139–40
   meditation, 153–54
   megadoses of vitamins and minerals, 132,
      143
   mind-body medicine, 153–54

complementary and alternative (*cont.*)
   multiple vitamin and mineral supplements, 134–35
   niacin, 135–36
   nopal (prickly pear cactus), 149
   omega-3 fatty acids, 140–41
   Russian tarragon (Tarralin), 151–52
   scientific data on, 132–33, 145–46
   vitamin C, 142–43
   vitamin E, 143–44
   glycation process, 35
   lifestyle interventions and, 34
   macrovascular, 48–55
   microvascular, 40–48
   prevention checklist, 55
   tests to detect and monitor, 36–40
complications of diabetes. *See also* heart disease; hypertension; vascular diseases
cost of diabetes care, 225–26
Coumadin, drug interactions with, 141, 144
C-reactive protein (CRP), 39–40, 49

DASH (Dietary Approaches to Stop Hypertension), 63–64, 76–82
DCCT (Diabetes Control and Complications Trial), 10–11, 44–45, 175–76
DiaBeta, 205
diabetes
   age at onset, 19
   cost of care, 225–26
   gestational diabetes, 15–16
   indications for testing, 32
   integrative management approach, 4, 9, 20
   lifestyle modifications, 30–31
   management obstacles, 11–12, 16–18
   signs and symptoms, 16, 29–30
   type 1 diabetes, 10–11, 12–13, 16
   type 2 diabetes, 11–13, 14–15, 16–18
   See also specific issues
Diabetes Forecast, Web address, 222
Diabetes Prevention Program. *See* DPP (Diabetes Prevention Program)
Diabinese (chlorpropamide), 205
diet. *See* menu plans; nutritional guidelines; recipes
Dietary Approaches to Stop Hypertension (DASH), 63–64, 76–82
Dietary Reference Intakes (DRIs), 131–32
dietary supplements. *See* complementary and alternative medicine (CAM)
digestion problems, 91
dining out, 76, 78–79, 108, 109

doctors, 189–90, 195–96
DPP (Diabetes Prevention Program), 17, 30, 63–64, 68–76, 157, 165–68
DPP-4 (dipeptidyl peptidase-IV) inhibitors, 210
DRIs (Dietary Reference Intakes), 131–32
drugs
   ACE (angiotensin converting enzymes) inhibitors, 45, 53
   Actoplus Met (pioglitazone + metformin), 208
   Actos (pioglitazone), 208–9
   alpha-blockers, 54
   alpha-glucosidase inhibitors, 207–8
   Amaryl (glimepiride), 205
   anticonvulsants, 47
   ARBs (angiotensin receptor blockers), 45, 53
   aspirin, 51, 144
   Avandamet (rosiglitazone + metformin), 208–9
   Avandaryl (rosiglitazone + glimepiride), 208
   Avandia (rosiglitazone), 32, 208–9
   beta-blockers, 53–54
   biguanides, 207
   bile acid resins, 50
   blood thinners, interactions with, 153
   Byetta (exenatide), 210–11
   calcium channel blockers, 54
   cholesterol-lowering, 50, 135
   combination therapy, 212–13
   Coumadin, interactions with, 141, 144
   DiaBeta, 205
   Diabinese (chlorpropamide), 205
   DPP-4 (dipeptidyl peptidase-IV) inhibitors, 210
   Duetact (pioglitazone + sulfonylurea glimepiride), 208–9
   efficacy of, to monitor, 213–14
   fibrates, 50
   Galvus (vildagliptin), 210
   glibenclamide, 140
   glucagon emergency kits, 215–16
   Glucophage (metformin), 17, 30–31, 207
   Glucotrol (glipizide), 138, 205
   Glynase, 205
   Glyset (miglitol), 208
   for hypertension, 53–54
   hypoglycemia side effect, 206, 214–16
   incretins, 2
   interactions, to avoid, 216
   Januvia (sitagliptin), 210
   meglitinides, 205–6

Micronase (glyburide), 205
new treatments, 210–12
Niaspan (niacin), 135–36
Orinase (tolbutamide), 205
pain reliever, topical, 47
Prandin (repaglinide), 205–6
Precose (acarbose), 208
reducing need for, 158–59
Rezulin (troglitazone), 30–31
secretagogues, 205–6
selective cholesterol-absorption
    inhibitors, 50
serotonin and norepinephrine reuptake
    inhibitor, 47
Starlix (nateglinide), 205–6
statins, 50, 135
sulfonylureas, 84, 205
Symlin (pramlintide acetate), 211–12
thiazide diuretics, 54
thiazolidinediones, 208–9
traditional treatments, 204–9
tricyclics, 47
value of, 203–4
vitamin therapy, 50
See also insulin therapy
Duetact (pioglitazone + sulfonylurea
    glimepiride), 208–9

electrocardiogram, 38
endothelial dysfunction, 142
exenatide (Byetta), 210–11
exercise
    benefits, 27–28, 156–60
    with diabetes complications, 168–71
    exercise specialists, 191
    guidelines, 27–28, 164–68
    injury treatment, 243–44
    with insulin therapy, 171–73
    lifestyle activity, 164, 167
    motivation for, 173–74
    preparation for, 160–61
    stretches, 241–43
    types of, 161–64
exercise stress test, 38–39
eye disease, 40–44, 168–69

fad diets, 87–88
family risk factors, 13, 14, 25
fat, body. See obesity
fats, blood. See cholesterol levels
fats, dietary, 27, 66–68, 69–73, 81
fenugreek supplements, 147
fiber, dietary, 61–62, 64, 65–66
fibrates, 50

food. See menu plans; nutritional guide-
    lines; recipes
Food Guide Pyramid, Web address, 69
foot care, 47–48

Galvus (vildagliptin), 210
garlic, 152–53
gastroparesis, 91
gestational diabetes, 15–16
GFR (glomerular filtration rate), 38
ginseng supplements, 150
glibenclamide, 140
glimepiride (Amaryl), 205
glipizide (Glucotrol), 138, 205
glucagon emergency kits, 215–16
Glucophage (metformin), 17, 30–31, 207
glucose. See blood sugar; blood sugar testing
Glucotrol (glipizide), 138, 205
glyburide (Micronase), 205
glycated hemoglobin test (A1c), 3, 37,
    184–85, 214
glycation process, 35
glycemic control. See blood sugar; blood
    sugar testing
glycemic index, 64, 86–87
glycemic response to exercise, 171–73
Glynase, 205
Glyset (miglitol), 208
gymnema sylvestre supplements, 147–48

HDL cholesterol. See cholesterol levels
heart disease
    blood lipid levels and, 48–49
    exercise and, 159, 171
    intensive insulin therapy and, 11, 176
    metabolic syndrome and, 16, 21–22
    screening for, 49
    signs of, 167–68
    treatment and management, 49–52
    weight loss and, 15
hemoglobin A1c test, 3, 37, 184–85,
    214
herbal supplements. See botanical extract
    supplements
high blood pressure. See hypertension
hunger management, 76
hyperglycemia, 12
hyperinsulinemia, 22
hypertension
    complications, 11, 52, 56
    DASH diet, 63–64
    drug interactions, 141
    drugs for, 45, 53–54
    exercise and, 159, 171

hypertension (*cont.*)
    metabolic syndrome and, 23, 28
    prevention, 52
hypoglycemia, 206, 214–16

impaired glucose tolerance (prediabetes),
    14, 16–17, 28–33
implantable continuous glucose monitors,
    179–81
incretins, 2
insulin
    blood glucose and, 12
    carbohydrate counting and, 82–83
    deficiency, 12
    hyperinsulinemia, 22
    low-fiber foods and, 61–62
    overweight and, 22–23, 91
    resistance, 12–13, 22–23
insulin therapy
    blood sugar monitoring, 223
    delivery systems, 220–24
    exercise and, 171–73
    intensive regimen, 11, 176
    plan, 222–23
    types, 218–19
    value of, 3, 217–18
    for visually impaired, 222
ivy gourd supplements, 148–49

Januvia (sitagliptin), 210
juvenile onset diabetes (type 1), 10–11,
    12–13, 16

ketoacidosis, 13
ketone testing, 184
kidney disease (nephropathy), 44–45,
    169
Kleefstra, Nanne, 138

LDL cholesterol. *See* cholesterol levels
libido, 56
lifestyle activity, 164, 167
lifestyle modifications. *See* exercise; nutri-
    tional guidelines
lipids, blood. *See* cholesterol levels

macrovascular complications, 48–55. *See
    also* heart disease; hypertension
magnesium supplements, 139–40
meal replacements, 87–89
Medicare coverage, 226
medications. *See* drugs
meditation, 153–54
meglitinides, 205–6

menu plans
    away-from-home strategies, 108–9
    day-by-day menus, 93–107
    guidelines, 93
    quick and easy meal ideas, 107
    See also nutritional guidelines; recipes
metabolic syndrome
    cardiometabolic risk factors, 21–23
    diagnosis, 23–25
    treatment, 26–28
metformin (Glucophage), 17, 30–31, 207
microalbuminuria, 38, 44
Micronase (glyburide), 205
miglitol (Glyset), 208
mind-body exercise, 163–64
mind-body medicine, 153–54
mineral supplements. *See* complementary
    and alternative medicine (CAM)
monitoring of blood sugar. *See* blood sugar
    testing
monitoring of complications, 36–40
monitoring of treatment, 213–14. *See also*
    record keeping

nateglinide (Starlix), 205–6
National Institutes of Health, Web ad-
    dresses, 153, 154
natural remedies. *See* complementary and
    alternative medicine (CAM)
nephropathy (kidney disease), 44–45, 169
neuropathy (nerve damage), 45–48, 91,
    169–71
niacin supplements, 135–36
Niaspan (niacin), 135–36
nopal supplements, 149
nutritional guidelines
    alcohol consumption, 84
    artificial sweeteners, 85
    business-lunch strategies, 108
    calorie reduction for weight loss, 73–74
    carbohydrate counting, 82–83
    carbohydrates, 64
    dairy foods, 80
    DASH (Dietary Approaches to Stop
    Hypertension), 63–64, 76–82
    diet foods, 86
    for digestion problems, 91
    DPP (Diabetes Prevention Program),
    63–64, 68–76
    DRIs (Dietary Reference Intakes),
    131–32
    eating behavior, 74–75
    fad diets, 87–88
    fat reduction, 69–73

fats and oils, 81
Food Guide Pyramid, 69
fruits, 80
hunger management, 76
meal replacements, 87–89
meats, poultry, and fish, 80
milk and milk products, 80
motivation, 90–91
nuts, seeds, and legumes, 81
protein, 45, 80
regular weighing, 74
restaurant meals, 76, 78–79, 108, 109
servings and food choices, 70–71, 77–82
slip-ups, 89
sodium, 28, 81
stress management to cope with changes,
    89–90
travel and vacation strategies, 109
unprocessed and low-fat foods, 61–62
vegetables, 77–80
weighing and measuring of foods, 83–84
whole grains, 77
See also menu plans; recipes
nutritional supplements. See complemen-
    tary and alternative medicine
    (CAM)

obesity
    abdominal fat, 22–23, 165
    as risk factor, 3, 15, 91
omega-3 fatty acid supplements, 140–41
oral glucose tolerance test (OGTT), 24–25
oral medications. See drugs
organ transplants, exercise and, 171
Orinase (tolbutamide), 205
outside support. See support team
overweight. See obesity

pancreas, 12, 220
payment assistance for diabetes care,
    225–26
physical activity. See exercise
physicians, 189–90, 195–96
Pilates, 163–64
pioglitazone (Actos), 208–9
pioglitazone + metformin (Actoplus Met),
    208
pioglitazone + sulfonylurea glimepiride
    (Duetact), 208–9
pramlintide acetate (Symlin), 211–12
Prandin (repaglinide), 205–6
Precose (acarbose), 208
prediabetes, 14, 16–17, 28–33
pregnancy, 15–16, 42, 84

prickly pear cactus supplements, 149
protein, dietary, 64–65
proteinuria (protein in urine), 38

recipes
  beef
    Beefsteak with Tomato-Orange Salsa,
        121
    Shepherd's Pie with Sweet Potato
        Topping, 120–21
  breakfasts
    Apple Smoothie, 111
    Broiled Grapefruit, 113
    Oat Bran Bread French Toast, 113–14
    Oat Bran Muffins, 114
    Oatmeal with Fruit, 112–13
    Raspberry Smoothie, 111
    Strawberry-Orange Smoothie, 112
    Tofu Colada, 112
  chicken
    Chicken Parmigiana, 123–24
    Chicken Wild Rice Salad with Mango,
        126
  desserts
    Rice Pudding, 129–30
    Strawberries in Balsamic Vinegar, 129
    Sweet Potato Custard, 130
  fish and seafood
    Baked Tuna Steaks with Peppers and
        Mushrooms, 121–22
    Fish in Spicy Tomato Sauce, 123
    Oven "Fried" Fish, 121
    Salmon and Vegetable Salad, 124–25
    Shrimp and Rice Salad, 125–26
    Tuna Niçoise Salad, 125
  salads, main dish
    Chicken Wild Rice Salad with Mango,
        126
    Salmon and Vegetable Salad, 124–25
    Shrimp and Rice Salad, 125–26
    Tuna Niçoise Salad, 125
  side dishes
    Baked Sweet Potato Fries, 128
    Braised Red Cabbage with Apple, 127
    Sautéed Broccoli and Garlic, 128–29
    Scallion Corn Bread, 127–28
  snacks
    Avocado and Tomato Salsa, 110–11
    Eggplant Dip, 110
  soups
    Black Bean Soup, 115
    Butternut Squash and Orange Soup,
        116–17
    Creamy Broccoli Soup, 116

vegetarian main dishes
    Bell Pepper Lasagna, 118–19
    Curried Garbanzo Beans, 117–18
    Potato Kale Frittata, 119
    Two-Minute Burritos, 117
record keeping
    blood sugar, 223
    food consumption, 71
    physical activity, 165–66
    treatment log, 196–99
    weight, 74
remedies, natural. *See* complementary and
    alternative medicine (CAM)
repaglinide (Prandin), 205–6
restaurant meals, 76, 78–79, 108, 109
retinopathy, 40–44, 168–69
Rezulin (troglitazone), 30–31
rosiglitazone (Avandia), 32, 208–9
rosiglitazone + glimepiride (Avandaryl), 208
rosiglitazone + metformin (Avandamet),
    208–9
Russian tarragon supplements, 151–52

secretagogues, 205–6
selective cholesterol-absorption inhibitors,
    50
self-monitoring. *See* blood sugar testing
serotonin and norepinephrine reuptake
    inhibitor, 47
serum creatinine test, 37–38
sexual performance, 56
signs and symptoms of diabetes, 16, 29–30
sitagliptin (Januvia), 210
smoking, 3, 28, 57
Starlix (nateglinide), 205–6
statins, 50, 135–36
strength training, 163, 164–65
stress management, 89–90, 154
stroke, 55
sugar, blood. *See* blood sugar; blood sugar
    testing
sugar-free foods, 85
sulfonylureas, 84, 205
supplements. *See* complementary and
    alternative medicine (CAM)
support team
    choice of professionals, 188–89
    diabetes educators, 190
    dietitians, 190–91
    doctors, 189–90, 195–96
    education programs, 192
    exercise specialists, 191
    as interdisciplinary approach, 187–88
    Internet services, 194–95

mental health counselors, 192
    payment assistance, 225–26
    pharmacists, 191–92
    support groups, 192–94
    to work with, 196–99
Symlin (pramlintide acetate), 211–12
symptoms of diabetes, 16, 29–30
syndrome X. *See* metabolic syndrome

tai chi, 163–64
Tarralin supplements, 151–52
thiazide diuretics, 54
thiazolidinediones, 208–9
thyroid function test, 37
Tolbutamide (Orinase), 205
tricyclics, 47
triglycerides. *See* cholesterol levels
troglitazone (Rezulin), 30–31
type 1 diabetes, 10–11, 12–13, 16
type 2 diabetes, 11–13, 14–15, 16–18

UKPDS (United Kingdom Prospective
    Diabetes Study), 11, 35–36, 44–45,
    175–76, 204
urine testing, 38, 183–84

vascular diseases.
    endothelial dysfunction, 142
    exercise and, 159, 170
    gastroparesis, 91
    high-risk category, 3
    intensive insulin therapy and, 11, 176
    intermittent claudication, 170
    nephropathy, 44–45, 169
    neuropathy, 45–48, 169–71
    retinopathy, 40–44, 168–69
    stroke, 55
    See also heart disease; hypertension
vildagliptin (Galvus), 210
vitamin supplements. *See* complementary
    and alternative medicine (CAM)
vitamin therapy, prescription, 50

waist-to-hip ratio, 24
weighing schedule, 74
weight loss
    alcohol consumption and, 84
    benefits, 31
    calorie reduction for, 73–74
    with exercise, 159
    meal replacements for, 87–89
    in treatment of metabolic syndrome, 27

yoga, 163–64